How Sadness Survived

the evolutionary basis of depression

Dr Paul Keedwell

BSc MB ChB MRCPsych

Radcliffe Publishing
Oxford • New York

Radcliffe Publishing Ltd
18 Marcham Road
Abingdon
Oxon OX14 1AA
United Kingdom

www.radcliffe-oxford.com
Electronic catalogue and worldwide online ordering facility.

British Library Cataloguing in Publication Data

A catalogue record for this book is available from the British Library.

ISBN-10 1 84619 013 4
ISBN-13 978 1 84619 013 1

Typeset by Ann Buchan (Typesetters), Middlesex, UK
Printed and bound by TJI Digital, Padstow, Cornwall

Contents

SECTION 1
Genes, disease and depression: busting myths

SECTION 2
The war of depression: an ancient human condition or a modern malaise?

SECTION 3
What has depression ever done for us?

To Michael James Keedwell

About the author

Dr Paul Keedwell is an Honorary Consultant Psychiatrist at the Mood Disorders Clinic, Maudsley Hospital, London and Lecturer in the Neuroscience of Emotion at the Institute of Psychiatry, London. He has published a significant body of work on the neurobiology of depression. He has a long held interest in communicating science to the general public, including some freelance work for BBC Radio Science. He continues to write for both the general and academic press. In his limited spare time he explores his love of architecture, movies, literature and music.

Acknowledgements

This work owes a debt to influential authors in the field of evolutionary psychology including Paul Gilbert, DM Buss, Randolph Nesse and Jonathon Price. It also owes a debt to those psychologists and neurologists who laid the foundations for this ever-growing field: Florence Goodenough, John Bowlby, Paul MacClean, Paul Ekman and Edward O Wilson. Many thanks to all who had the patience to read through my manuscript and give me some guidance on its direction, including my friends Justine, Tim, Kelly and Ollie, my old school master John Denness, my mother, Angela, my late father Michael, my brother James, my sister Alice, Leyla and Steph at the Marsh Agency, Lisa, Paula and Gillian at Radcliffe, and all those who have been involved in the production of this book who I have not mentioned.

Introduction

It is often said that depression is a modern Western malaise. There are so many pressures on us today, and we have not evolved to deal with them. The media fills our heads with unfulfilled dreams and the need for perfection in all aspects of our lives. We seem to get our goals in the wrong order of priority – putting working for a new car ahead of spending time with the family. In our childhoods we are more likely to be neglected by our busy professional parents, or come from broken homes. We have become wage slaves, trapped in jobs or marriages we detest. We don't support each other, we live apart from our wider families, some of us are poor, alienated and forgotten, some of us are exposed to crime and prejudice on a daily basis, and some of us, although privileged, have more leisure time to mull things over, ruminate on the illusory world that celebrity culture has provided us. We turn to sex, drugs and rock and roll for their short term antidepressant qualities. We move from little high to little high with long periods of misery in between. And then, gradually or suddenly 20–25% of us fall victim of a state more pervasive and more handicapping than ordinary misery – the illness of major depression. Mind and body take on an involuntary collapse, thoughts slow down, energy fades; chasing the modern media-led illusion gives way to moribund negativity, social withdrawal and introspection. Things can get really bad. We can stop sleeping and lose weight. We might even think about ending our lives. We can't get the same joy from our favourite song, a beautiful sunset or a chocolate cake. Normally we would love chocolate cake. We can't cope so well at work, and ordinary housework seems like a huge struggle. But slowly, after some weeks or months we seem to come out of it, grateful that we no longer feel so awful and resolving never to feel so awful again.

But we do not have time to be depressed in the modern world. It is extremely inconvenient. How on earth can we pay our mortgages and keep our demanding partners? There is no time for slowing down and taking stock. So, we have developed new technologies – antidepressant medications – that will bring things to an end swiftly, so we can get back to earning a living and consuming. When you develop a technology it is important to develop a disease to go with it – the depressive disorder. There is no doubt that depression is an illness, and it can be so severe that it can lead to loss of life, or we can become stuck in depression, but most of the time depression does not lead to permanent harm, and its course is self-limiting, providing there is no ongoing stress around to perpetuate it. Most episodes of depression that are observed in the general population, or in people attending their family doctor, tend to get better within 12 months, often without antidepressant treatment.[1,2] Psychiatrists frequently forget this.

Psychiatrists tend to see the more severe 'melancholic' forms of depression which can lead to weight loss, stuporous inactivity, psychotic symptoms (like hearing critical voices), attempted suicide, and admission to hospital. These varieties of depression are rare. They can become chronic and tend to recur – up to 16% of hospitalised depressed patients may still be depressed several years later. This book will focus on the mild to moderate types that most people experience, and try to get a handle on why they are so common.

The notion of depression as a disease has been reinforced and perpetuated by biologists, psychiatrists and pharmaceutical companies, all of whom have a vested interest, consciously or unconsciously, in the clinical perspective. Although technological advances in antidepressant treatments have undoubtedly been responsible for the alleviation of much suffering, strict adherence to a medical model may be preventing a more complete understanding of why we humans are so susceptible to depression. It may also be engendering a sense of powerlessness in sufferers or ex-sufferers. What so commonly goes along with the disease model is the implication that the condition is quite special, quite unusual, and probably due to some permanent and rare weakness of brain biology, perhaps due to a genetic defect. The only solution, therefore, is chemical.

But it is a complete nonsense to say that a condition that will affect at least 20% of men and 25% of women in their lifetimes is unusual. It is quite plainly common. A larger proportion of the population will become depressed if they belong to a 'high risk' group – like the poor and socially isolated. Addiction to drugs or alcohol also increases the risk. A survey carried out by the European Neuropsychopharmacological Society (ECNP) suggests that the risk might be even higher in Europe than these figures, derived from the USA, suggest (different methods and definitions were used).

Although these figures are based on reasonably careful surveys, there is much scope for disagreement over the real rate of depression, at least in Western Society: some researchers say depression is more common than this; some say it is less common. I take the former position, for several reasons: Firstly, we tend to re-label depression as grief or 'heartbreak' because of the stigma associated with admitting that we are 'depressed'. Freud highlighted the similarities between loss reactions and depression over half a century ago in his book 'Mourning and Melancholia'. Secondly, depression can be difficult to detect in ourselves, particularly at the start of the illness, and especially if its onset is insidious. Thirdly, memory biases can occur in people if they are asked to recall previous episodes of depression. When we are functioning normally, we tend to think that we have been happier than is actually the case. We can overlook times when we have been depressed.

The reason for this may be cultural, but it is also possible that depression is not just an accident of culture, but a condition that has evolved for a functional reason – to give us new and more radical insights. Robert Frost was right when he said that taking the path less trodden can make all the difference in life,[3] but only when we have the right attributes to take that route; it is only true if we are not labouring under some illusion, sacrificing our own needs to please others, or bringing emotional problems, arising in the past, to bear on decisions in the present.

This war of depression – between the view that it is enlightening and the view that it is hindering – has raged for a long time. The truth is that depression is multifaceted: it can lead to great insights and achievements, as well as great tragedies. Although Van Gogh was driven to suicide, the depression of the philosopher John Stuart Mill seemed to him to be helpful in retrospect. Mill wrote 'On Utilitarianism' at the age of 19 and became depressed at the age of 21. Upon recovery he confessed that the experience had taught him an important lesson – that he should not sacrifice his social and emotional development to intellectual ambition.[4] More than two thousand years ago Socrates had warned of the same danger: melancholia was thought to be a consequence of rigorous philosophising. However, Aristotle believed it to be a state of immense moral and spiritual value because of the insights it could bring. At the higher level of intellectual debate, depression was often regarded as a gift of the Gods.

So, depression may not be all bad. Rather than being a defect it could be some kind of defence, and represent a part of what it means to be human. Could it be that it defends us against the tendency to deny our true needs and brings these needs more into focus?

The eminent biologist Lewis Wolpert wrote bravely and eloquently on his own experience of depression, which was quite severe in nature.[5] He regarded it as a 'malignant' dysregulation of ordinary sadness – a unique form of blackness brought about by a disturbance of the biology which normally regulates our sad feelings, and spirals out of control. However, if all depression is a disease – where sadness spirals out of control – we might conclude that a great many brains are poorly designed. Why don't depressed people just bounce back from adversity? Does depression occur because our higher brain centres have become over-evolved? The more complex a system becomes, the more likely it is to go wrong: There might be a poor junction between the recently evolved intellectual brain and the older, mood-regulating brain, for example.

Wolpert's views are consistent with perfectly reasonable explanations for why depression exists commonly in humans which have nothing to do with inherent usefulness: it may be a by-product of something more useful but ubiquitous, like language, or the capacity for day-to-day sadness. Alternatively, *or in addition*, our brains may have been perfectly adapted to the ancient environment but now seem badly designed for the modern one.

If we can show that depression has persisted since ancient times, this makes the idea that depression is potentially helpful more tenable. If depression *has* persisted one possible explanation is that, in most individuals, the short term pain led to longer term gain. This could still be true, even in the 'developed' world, although considerations like earning a wage and paying a mortgage tend to make us focus on the short-term, and may make us ignore the lessons of depression. A recently published follow-up study of depression, conducted in Holland, suggests that depression is indeed helpful in the longer term: researchers were surprised to discover that people seemed to cope better with life's trials after depression than they were doing before its onset.[2]

This report was based on the Netherlands Mental Health Survey and Incidence Study (NEMESIS), a general population survey of Dutch people aged 18–64 years. It was conducted in three waves: 1996, 1997, and 1999. In the group as a whole, averaged ratings of vitality, psychological health, social and leisure activities, occupational performance and general health all significantly *improved* upon recovery from depression compared to functioning *prior to* the depression. A minority of individuals got worse after a depressive episode, mostly in the realms of general health, vitality, and physical functioning. However, much to the authors' surprise, severity of depression, and availability of treatment, were not significant predictors of functional decline. Rather, the most important contributions to increased disability after depression were factors that were not directly to do with the depression itself, like social isolation (pre-dating the depression), and *co-existing conditions*, including drug misuse, anxiety disorder or physical illness. Furthermore, if these people were bringing the average down, this meant that the majority, that did not have these co-existing problems, had *even larger* improvements in func-tioning, particularly psychological, occupational and social functioning, than the averages suggested.

The second section of this book considers the evidence for depression persisting and this lays the groundwork for considering why depression might have persisted in Sections 3 and 4. Could it be that depression was in some ways beneficial to us, as the NEMESIS study suggests? What were the situations in the lives of the early *Homo sapiens* that might have shaped our capacities for sadness and depression? The media obsession with promoting happiness has led to a neglect of what Professor Randolpe Nesse, a pioneer of the evolutionary approach to psychology, has called 'diagonal psychology': a consideration of the *dangers* of unwarranted positive states and the *benefits* of negative emotions.[6] So, for example, depression might be better for us than blind optimism. Blind optimism could lead to frustration, exhaustion, injury, or even death.

There are important implications for how we should prevent or re-act to depression (our winter evergreen) and how we might view the condition in a more constructive way.

References

1   Barkow K, Maier W, Ustun TB, Gansicke M, Wittchen HU, Heun R. Risk factors for depression at 12-month follow-up in adult primary health care patients with major depression: an international prospective study. *Journal of Affective Disorders* 2003; **76**: 157–169.

2   Buist-Bouwman MA, Ormel J, de Graaf R, Vollebergh WAM. Functioning after a major depressive episode: complete or incomplete recovery? *Journal of Affective Disorders* 2004; **82**: 363–371.

3   I have paraphrased from Frost's famous poem 'The Road Not Taken', which was published in 1916 in the collection 'Mountain Interval'. See Lathem E (Editor). *The Poetry of Robert Frost*. London: Vintage books. 2001.

4   Capaldi, Nicholas. *John Stuart Mill: A Biography*. Cambridge, 2004.

5   Wolpert L. *Malignant sadness. The anatomy of depression. London*: Faber and Faber, 2001.

6   Nesse RM. Natural selection and the elusiveness of happiness. *Philos Trans R Soc Lond B Biol Sci* 2004; **359**: 1333–1347.

Crucial definitions

Sadness

A transient state of low mood that we all experience from time to time, following defeats and losses. There is a relative paralysis of mind and a retardation of the body: one's posture is slumped and there is a feeling of exhaustion and deflation. The down-turned mouth and furrowed brow are universal expressions of sadness.

Depression

A condition characterised by unremitting sadness, reduced energy, and anhedonia (*an* 'lack of', *hedonia* 'pleasure'), lasting for at least two weeks (but usually months), and usually triggered by stress. Anhedonia, referring more specifically to a loss of pleasure in reaction to what were, formerly, rewarding activities or events, is a core feature. Depression, therefore, is not alleviated by activities that might have been enjoyable in the past. There is a variable reduction in the capacity to carry out work or engage socially with others. Mental energies are impaired, as well as bodily responses, leading to poor concentration, absent-mindedness and vacillation. Curiously, the mood can also affect the content of thought, leading to feelings of helplessness, worthlessness (low self-esteem), and even hopelessness about the future. There is a tendency to look back on life and minimise successes but magnify failures. However, milder depression is thought by many to be associated with 'depressive realism' – a removal of the falsely positive bias engaged in by non-depressed people, whereby they believe they have more control over personal outcomes than is actually the case.[1] (More about this later). Biological functions of sleep, sex drive and appetite may be affected in all severities of depression.

Depression is associated with the depletion of a group of chemical messengers called monoamines (which include serotonin, noradrenaline and dopamine). These chemicals are found in areas of the brain that are crucial for the control of mood, concentration, drive, sexual activity, appetite, sleep, and pleasure. It is thought that the depletion occurs due to stress but it is poorly understood why the depletion persists for weeks or months before the body starts to replenish itself. Once depression starts it is like a runaway train. It will take its own course, and it is hard to fight it with more positive thoughts and behaviours, although this can help to alleviate the painful symptoms. In milder forms of depression it is still possible to function at work, do the housework, engage in leisure activities and socialise. In moderately severe forms disability is evident in all these domains, although some people may be good at hiding it.

'Endogenous' depression
A controversial term for a type of depression that is thought to be triggered by internal biological (brain) events rather than significant life events. It tends to be associated with more severe slowing of the body and mind, and is thought to be highly genetic in origin. However, it is difficult to prove that it is not brought on by the cumulative effect of lots of minor stresses.

Melancholia
An ancient term which referred to all types of depression but which is now used by some psychiatrists to describe the more severe and incapacitating forms of the condition, with marked biological symptoms of reduced sleep and weight loss, and stronger associations with suicide. Individuals with melancholia find it almost impossible to work and socialise, and may have intense suicidal thoughts. Most cases of depression are less severe and sufferers continue to work and socialise on a superficial level, but with less engagement and enjoyment. They tire more easily but do not grind to a halt. The evolutionary argument is probably strongest for non-melancholic forms of depression, and these are the forms that I will concentrate on.

Grief
A reaction to loss, characterised by the sequential responses of shock (and numbness), denial, anger, depression, then acceptance. The depression phase can be prolonged, leading to diagnostic confusion with the above.

Pathological grief

Prolonged or severe grief. It occurs when ongoing life difficulties, the circumstances of the death, or individual personality traits, cause someone to be 'stuck' in one of the stages before 'acceptance'.[2] There is no consensus on how long people should take to pass through the different stages, causing diagnostic confusion with the above, and with depressive illness.

References

1   Aloy, L. B. and Abramson, L. Y. (1988). Depressive realism: Four theoretical perspectives. In L. B. Aloy (Ed.), *Cognitive processes in depression* (pp. 223–265). New York: Guilford.

2   Parkes, C. M. (1998). *Bereavement: studies of grief in adult life* (3rd ed.). London: Penguin.

The hypothesis

The genetic and biological blueprint for grief and mild to moderate depression is common, ancient and universal, and occurs in all mammals. The human brain's capacity for grief and depression has persisted because, *on average*, the advantages of these unpleasant states of mind have outweighed, or at least equalled, the disadvantages in the environment of our ancestors. Depression may still have the potential to help us in the modern day, provided we understand its meaning.

Why didn't I kneel more deeply to accept you, inconsolable sisters
And, surrendering, lose myself in your loosened hair?
How we squander our hours of pain.
How we gaze beyond them into the bitter duration
To see if they have an end. Though they are our winter foliage,
Our dark evergreen, our season in our inner year.
Not only a season in time – but our place and settlement,
Our, foundation, soil and home.

*'Tenth Elegy', translated by Stephen Mitchell,
from THE SELECTED POETRY OF RAINER MARIA RILKE
by Rainer Maria Rilke, translated by Stephen Mitchell,
copyright ©1982 by Stephen Mitchell.
Used by permission of Random House, Inc.*

Genes, disease and depression: busting myths

Myth 1: We come into the world as a blank slate: how we think and feel is determined only by experience

Myth 1 is the 'standard social science' model of thinking and emotion.[1] It is just as wrong as saying that everything we think, do and feel is determined by our genes. The mind is the last battle ground for these two polarised positions. Although general medicine ditched this false dichotomy years ago – realising that human anatomy and physiology, health and disease, were all a product of an interaction between both genes *and* environment, psychology has been struggling to find this middle ground when it comes to defining both mental health and mental illness. We seem reluctant to examine what parts of our minds are determined by evolution and what parts seem to be unique to the individual or his experiences. You could assert that this is because there are no fossils of human behaviour. However, for centuries now we have been documenting human behaviour in all contexts around the globe. Furthermore, there are traditional hunter–gatherer communities to examine in the present day, whose cultures might, to a certain extent, represent 'living fossils' of our ancestors, despite the influence of observers and the insidious seep of modern urban life. We can look for certain 'universals' of thinking and emotion which are common to all cultures. We can also examine the behaviour of other mammals from which we presume to have evolved.

So, this type of study, what we might call evolutionary psychology (EP), provides the middle ground between nature and nurture that a proper understanding of psychiatry and psychology requires. We have the capacity to learn and improve on what we started out with, but what we started out with was shaped by evolution and genetic variation. EP goes beyond examining the individual and starts to explore what it means to be human. In the language of the evolutionary psychologist, this equates to the difference between the 'proximate' and 'ultimate' causes of human conditions. A young woman might have a phobia of snakes that is so severe that even seeing pictures of the creatures in a book makes her heart pound and her throat turn dry with fear. The proximate cause might have been coming across a snake while hiking as a young girl. The ultimate cause, however, would be to do with her ancestors on the plains of Africa, and the impact that being bitten by a poisonous snake would have had on their survival (and hence the propagation of their genes). The eminent psychologist Martin Seligman demonstrated decades ago that we have an increased tendency to develop phobias of snakes (and spiders) over much more modern dangers, like guns. He called this phenomenon 'preparedness'.[2] Emotional 'programs' like these evolved over millennia and are not going to be modified quickly. Psychologically, we are still living in the caves.

Another influential psychologist called Garcia demonstrated how our ability to learn to avoid foods that make us ill several hours later, and after just one trial, does not conform to the idea that all human behaviour starts from a blank slate.[3] Before Garcia's experiments most psychologists were wedded to 'behaviourism', the scientific movement which seemed to be able to prove that all human learning conformed to certain rules – the rules of 'classical' or 'operant' conditioning. In summary, in order to learn, behaviour had to be closely paired in time with a consequence. Also, a negative consequence would need to occur several times before it extinguished a formally learned behaviour. Eating is normally rewarded with feeling satiated, and if a food tastes good we will not hesitate to eat it. However, if that food contains something noxious, and we later vomit as a result, we will immediately acquire a distaste for that particular food that lasts pretty much indefinitely. The evolutionary implications of this are clear – if you don't learn to associate the taste with illness after one trial, and some time after tasting the food, you will not live very long. Garcia proved this 'preparedness' for a unique type of learning in a laboratory experiment. He showed that he could make rats learn a distaste for sugary water by making them ill with radiation several hours later.

To give an example closer to depression, the proximate cause of grief is the death of a loved one, but the ultimate cause is to do with the importance that emotional bonds have played in the history of social mammals, and how grief might be an important way of processing and accepting a loss. It makes perfect sense, from an EP point of view, that the loss of an intimate partner should cause more distress than the loss of a remote relative, because the effect on reproductive success is more direct in the former case. Negative feelings initially help us to strive for the lost person, but if the loss is due to death the pining is futile, and we will need to go through the process of accepting the loss. The closeness that we had prior to the loss must be unlearned; otherwise we can not seek out new bonds that are important for propagating our genes.

Hence, to what degree evolution plays a role in our functioning today is the real question for EP, and the real question underlying this book. Different functions of the brain – like recognising a smile, fearing a snake, getting sexually aroused by the particular shape of a man or woman's body, manipulating a tool, solving a problem, and learning a language – have all been shaped by different evolutionary pressures, with some overlaps. These human capacities, coded for by a few or by many genes, some constant in shape and effect, some varying, will interact with each other and the environment, and will vary across the general population. On average they will have persisted because they gave the ancestors carrying those genes a competitive advantage over others – leading to a better share of resources and sexual partners, and hence giving the vessel of those genes the edge in terms of survival and reproductive success. Some complex but apparently inherent skills, like musical ability, seem at first glance to be difficult to explain in terms of evolution. Why should a concert pianist pass on his ability to his child? Environment is not enough to explain this alone – some people will be pushed into music classes from an early age but will never achieve the level of concert pianist. In the case of rare musical ability the gifted musician will have co-inherited a number of characteristics like good hand–eye coordination, optimal hearing, emotional sensitivity and good communication skills. In other words, musical ability is a pleasant by-product of more important skills that would have increased the reproductive success of our ancestors in the close-knit hunter–gatherer environments of their time.

A human quality that directly influenced differential reproductive success in a given environment is what Darwin coined an 'adaptation'. Qualities that are inherited alongside adaptations are by-products, or genetic 'fluff'.[4] The evolutionary psychologist's role is to identify which characteristics of the human mind are adaptations and which are fluff. So, when considering the ultimate cause of the common condition of depression we might conclude that it is just fluff, a consequence of the development of emotional sensitivity, empathy, language and other social aspects of intelligence. It is possible that you can not have these other human qualities without a tendency to experience depression.

On the other hand, depression may have directly influenced reproductive success because it led to some competitive advantage.

Myth 2: Evolutionary psychology implies that behaviour is under genetic control

EP is accused of genetic determinism – the proposition that genes and only genes determine and limit our successes and failures.[5] Although sociobiologists of the past might have taken up such an extreme position, EP at its best is sociobiology 'grown up' – it has absorbed all the evidence, which has emerged more recently, which confirms that psychological functioning is affected by both environment *and* genetics. Thus, EP has room to acknowledge that depression may have an ancient biological blueprint while also acknowledging that it may be on the increase due to modern cultural pressures. Both can be true at the same time. One aspect does not invalidate the other. In fact, modern theories of evolution recognise the phenomenon of genetic and cultural 'co-evolution', whereby changes in culture, like changes in the notion of beauty, lead to the selection of different genes for that culture, or when a new genetic mutation that allows for, say, the development of language, lead to cultural changes, which then make genes coding for social awareness more important, and so on.

Also, EP is the preferred model for exploring the idea that human conditions like depression may have been modified over time: depression may have become more malignant and more chronic in the last few centuries due to many major cultural shifts, although the evidence for this is lacking at present. An evolutionary perspective helps us to take in to account the following facts when thinking about prevention of depression:

- the human genome was selected in ancestral environments which were very different from the modern environment, at least in the developed world
- cultural development now occurs too quickly for genes to adapt, resulting in a split between our genes and our lifestyles
- this mismatch between biology and lifestyle can bring about illness, make illness worse, make an illness last longer, or change the nature of an illness.
- adaptations will always represent a balance between benefits and costs because they are never perfect. The erect human spine causes a lot of problems but it is interesting to speculate on the benefits that must have outweighed these costs. There is no reason why we

cannot speculate in the same way about psychology and behaviour. The brain is a physical structure, after all, and one that has been under the control of gene selection.

Myth 3: Evolutionary explanations for human psychology have no basis and can not be proved

EP is often attacked for coming up with fanciful, un-testable biological explanations for complex human behaviour. It is accused of making up 'just so stories', that can neither be proved nor refuted.[6] This is to belittle the honest process of hypothesis formation – the creation of a consistent, coherent theory, based on what we now know, that we may test in the future. [7] Darwin's original ideas were mere hypotheses, but they were consistent with the evidence at the time and they were held together by rational argument.[8] He was struck, like his predecessors, by the observation that animals, like the giraffe or woodpecker, seemed to be so well adapted to their environments, but he also noted the similarities between the structures of the hand, the flipper and the wing. Subsequently, more and more evidence emerged to support his view, so his ideas developed beyond a theory towards being accepted as a 'best fit' model in the world of science. Darwin is not criticised for developing a theory of how things might have been hundreds of thousands of years ago, based on what he recorded in the nineteenth century. Similarly, Noam Chomsky's conclusions on the universal rules of language, which led to his proposition that we had evolved a 'language acquisition device' (in other words we have certain rules of language structure *imprinted* in our brains which mean that we learn language much more quickly than would be possible just by trial and error), were based on a reasonable hypothesis and careful observation. He did not need to travel back in time.

So, returning to depression, the results of large-population follow-up surveys of children and young adults are being published in this millennium, which give new and exciting opportunities to test the possible utility of depression, because they can examine functioning in many areas of life – work, recreation, relationships – before, during and after a major depression, like the NEMESIS study carried out in Holland.[9] They will challenge the idea that evolutionary theories are not testable.

Myth 4: Depression must be a disease because it is unpleasant and undesirable

At first it seems absurd to consider that depression could be considered anything other than unhelpful, but this is due to social conditioning – what you could call the 'assumption of disease'. Major depression is considered a disease because it is socially undesirable, interferes with work efficiency, makes the sufferer feel ill, is associated with more physical illness, causes distress and is linked to suicide. Let me take each point in turn:

1. Although depression is often incompatible with functioning well at work, there is a difference between modern and ancestral environments that may make depression seem unhelpful in the urbanised world. Depression could still be helpful in other, more important ways following recovery, or it may have been adaptive in the past, but not now. Modern urban life might cause people to become 'trapped' in stressful situations, so that depression is perpetuated and becomes more severe. In the latter case, depression is not being allowed to function as perhaps it should (as a period of 'time out') and urbanisation is at fault, not the depression. Depression may have been shaped by urbanisation into something more severe and less helpful.
2. Depression is associated with subjective distress, but this does not imply disorder. The feeling of disgust is subjectively unpleasant, as is the process of vomiting, but no-one would doubt the survival value of these universal human capacities. In other words, unpleasant but instinctive mental reactions, just like the physical examples given above, could be defences rather than disorders. A fear of heights is unpleasant but it is understood to be protective. Similarly, the absence of fear in the face of possible injury or death is considered abnormal. It is equally possible to regard the absence of depression in reaction to certain life events as abnormal.
3. Depression is regarded as socially undesirable, but this does not imply an unhelpful process. People often withdraw from social contact when they have flu, or if they are grieving over a loss, but this is for a good reason. They want to recuperate before returning to the fold.
4. Feeling ill does not equate with disorder. A short term illness can lead to long term benefits. When we suffer a stomach illness after

food poisoning is this a disorder or a normal reaction? Would we consider a fever to be a normal or an abnormal reaction to infection? Similarly, should we consider depression to be an abnormal reaction to stress or loss?

The existence of severe melancholic depression (see definitions) does not necessarily effect depression's adaptiveness overall. A good analogy is the functioning of the immune system: The immune system works well most of the time but occasionally works against us. Mast cells are part of the immune system that work in the nasal passages and skin to protect us from invading 'foreign bodies', like grass pollen. For the majority, the mast cell reaction to grass pollen is proportionate. However, in a minority of people, there is a propensity for the hypersensitivity reaction that we call hay fever. Hay fever is inconvenient but not life-threatening. Rarer still are those people who have a very severe form of allergy known as anaphylaxis. Such people react to the allergenic substance, say shellfish, with angioedema (swelling of throat and larynx), and an asthma-type reaction in the lungs which can obstruct breathing. Extreme reactions can cause death within minutes. The bottom line is that the immune system is very useful to the large majority of us because otherwise we would be killed by any invading toxin. The fact that some people with extreme allergic reactions may die does not significantly affect the propagation of the genes controlling the immune system for the population of humans as a whole. So, it can be argued that severe clinical depression, like anaphylaxis, is a consequence of genetic variation. Human adaptations need only be helpful 'on average' for their genes to survive and propagate. We must also remember that the process of natural selection does not end with the present day. The most disabling types of depression may be bred out in the future.

Myth 5: Depression can not be regarded as helpful because it causes suicide

It is commonly said that depression lies behind most suicide, and therefore depression is a bad thing. National and international mental health organisations talk about the need to treat depression in order to get suicide figures down.[10] This perspective is fundamentally misguided because it fails to grasp the real relationship between society, depression and suicide.

Passive suicidal ideas – thoughts that life is not worth living, for example – *are* a reasonably common symptom of depression, but forming the genuine intention to die is an uncommon feature, and taking real steps to carry out suicide is rarer still.

It is commonly believed that anyone who takes his or her own life must be depressed. This is a fallacy and an oversimplification of reality. In fact only about 30% of suicides are committed during a depressive illness, and there are usually co-existing problems and social causes. Suicide is also importantly linked to schizophrenia, drug misuse, alcoholism, an impulsive or psychopathic personality, or a combination of all these problems.[11] Also, not all those who commit suicide have a mental disorder or illness. Surprisingly, only a quarter of people who commit suicide are under psychiatric care in the year before their death. Suicide is often regarded as an understandable reaction to having a chronic, painful and incurable illness. Suicide is also associated with being a member of a cult or holding extreme religious or political views (consider the Palestinian suicide bombers, or partners in the mass suicide pact in Waco, Texas). Some people who kill themselves for a political or religious cause, like the suicide bombers of Hamas, believe that their actions will be rewarded in the afterlife. From their perspective suicide is a rational choice, born out of strong religious beliefs and cultural allegiances. In a public debate at the Maudsley Hospital in London in 2001 it was proposed that the reaction of most Americans to the terrorist atrocity of 11 September was 'madder' than the acts of the Al Qaeda terrorists themselves. Following a far-reaching debate, those in favour of the motion won the final vote. It is a mistake to assign the label of madness to a group if their actions are understandable within a cultural context, even if that culture seems twisted and abhorrent. A person who dies in such an action firmly believes that he is a martyr, who will be rewarded in the afterlife by Allah. So, we can not imply that all suicides are committed by people of unbalanced mind. Very often the cause is cultural, or has a sociological explanation.

At a national level depression rates and suicide statistics often fail to match up. For example, a country like Iran has more depression than was previously thought to be the case – but relatively low rates of suicide.[12] This may be largely due to religious and cultural taboos, which not only prevent suicidal behaviour but distort official statistics. For example, in unclear cases coroners may choose, either deliberately or unconsciously, to record likely suicides as death by 'undetermined' cause in order to spare the added burden of shame on the bereaved

This was historically common practice in Ireland, and might still be a common practice in Portugal.[13] However, variations in suicide rates may reflect variations in levels of cumulative stress and differences in community values. The common denominator in most cases of suicide, including those associated with depression, is isolation or social adversity.

The absence of constraining social contacts is important, as reflected in indicators like divorce, the number of close friends, and loss of crucial significant others through bereavement. As important as stress and negative life events is the feeling that no-one cares if you live or die.[14] Hence, societies that have more cohesive communities may have lower rates of suicide than societies with a lot of segregation and fostering of independent aspirations to succeed. Durkheim, the eminent sociologist, explained suicide in terms of this kind of societal pathology, (which he called the 'anomic society'), rather than the pathology of the individual.[15] His focus was not on depression, but on the social conditions which breed isolation and despair. Such conditions would not have been common in the close knit groups of our ancestors, where there was a very strong sense of interdependence. These were the conditions in which depression evolved.

The modern phenomenon of 'entrapment' may combine with increasing isolation to cause an abnormally persistent or severe form of depression and other mental health problems, which then become associated with suicide. Entrapment is a term introduced by social scientists to describe the phenomenon of being trapped in a stressful situation. On an individual level, modern examples include the single mother with four young children and no support, or someone financially dependent on an exploitative employer. On a society level they include War and societies in transition. So, while the website of the Suicide Prevention department of World Health Organisation states that mental disorder is present in 90% of suicide cases (however they define 'disorder'), it then goes on to say that suicide results from 'many complex sociocultural factors and is more likely to occur particularly during periods of socioeconomic, family and individual crisis situations'. Hence social circumstances and cultural phenomena are the common mediating factors that drive both mental illness and suicide. Figure 1 shows this idea in diagrammatic form.

So, saying that a suicide is caused by depression is no more enlightening than saying that a death by heart attack was due to a blocked coronary artery. The heart attack was ultimately due to a

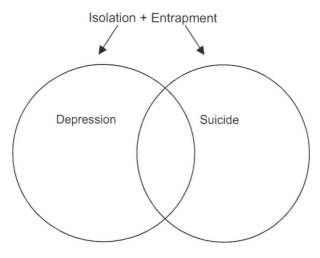

Figure 1 Suicide and depression

combination of an ancient instinct to eat calorific foods and a modern western lifestyle. Additional proximate causes would have been to do with chosen lifestyle, work demands and culturally sanctioned behaviours resulting in stress, lack of exercise, drinking alcohol to excess, or smoking. Similarly, an act of suicide might be tapping in to certain ultimate causes of depression, but in addition there will be the overlay of the social conditions of entrapment and isolation, leading to something different to just misery – a strong sense of hopelessness.

During a radio debate on the evolutionary theories of depression an argument was put forward for a 'fitness advantage' for human suicide.[16] It has been argued that if you are not productive yourself due to any kind of disability or illness, if you have reached a certain age, and pro-created, and if being alive puts a strain on the resources of those around you, it would be useful if you were to kill yourself and let your offspring get on with the job of propagating your genes. This is not such a strange theory if you consider how the life of a honey bee comes to an end. However, it does come from the extreme end of adaptationist theory. In my view, it is dangerous to try to posit a fitness advantage for a rare event. It is not justified. Otherwise you might suggest an evolutionary explanation for multiple sclerosis, or diabetes. In the UK in 2002, your risk of suicide was 0.015% if you were female, 0.043% if you were male.[17] So, it is a rare event in anyone's book. And while the rate of suicide is going down in the UK, according to the official statistics, the rate of depression is going up, suggesting a less than perfect relationship.

Recent research suggests that the neurobiology of depression and suicide are distinct and separate. Gambling tests (the IOWA gambling task is often used) suggest that people with a history of depression but no suicide attempts perform better, i.e. win more money, than those with a history of suicide attempts.[18] This is thought to be due to a greater tendency in the suicidal group to act impulsively. These tests are being combined with neuro-imaging to see if differences can be found in blood flow to different parts of the brain.

Depression and suicide seem to have different patterns of inheritance within a family tree. The Amish communities of the *United States* and *Ontario, Canada*, who are known for their plain dress and limited use of modern devices such as *automobiles* and *electricity*, separate themselves from mainstream society for religious reasons. The result of this isolation is a well defined gene pool and as a result the genetic determinants of many human characteristics have been examined using the Amish. Studies on suicidal behaviour reveal that the family histories of suicide separate from the family histories of depression. In other words, there might be a genetic predisposition to suicide which is separate from the genes coding for depression. Depressed people commonly have thoughts of suicide but mostly stop short of committing the act. Self-preservation instincts usually take over, even in the depths of despair. Suicide 'completers' seem to have an impulsive aspect to their personalities, which propel them towards the final act. A greater propensity to express anger and emotional instability is also thought to be linked to suicide. It should also be noted, when thinking about how suicide relates to depression, that although women experience more depression than men, suicide is overwhelmingly more common in men than in women. This can be partly, but not entirely, explained by the fact that men tend to use more violent and lethal methods than women.

To sum up, depression is unfairly 'blamed' for suicide, which deserves a more sophisticated sociological explanation. Those severe forms of depression that may have a more direct association with suicide are rare, and are outside the scope of this book.

Because the dangers of depression are sometimes very apparent – like suicide, or weight loss, or psychotic symptoms (experiencing hallucinations or delusions) an assumption is often made that *all* depression is unhelpful. 'Mistakes' accompany the average functioning of most human characteristics, due to genetic variation. Depression is probably no exception. Most depressive illnesses are of mild to moderate severity, and occur as a reaction to stress. Although the risk of suicide in a severely depressed person must be taken seriously, most suicides are not carried out in the midst of a depressive illness. Many suicides are erroneously and retrospectively attributed to depression, while social factors are overlooked.

Myth 6: Depression makes us more prone to other diseases

An association does not prove a cause.

A large body of research has suggested that depression lowers our resistance to infection, by suppressing certain parts of the immune system.[19] Other research suggests that depression increases our risk of suffering from conditions like heart disease, or increases the severity of these diseases following their onset and leads to premature death. These assertions, if true, support the disease model and challenge the 'depression-as-adaptation' idea.

Our natural 'killer' cells help us to kill other body cells that have been infected by viruses. One study showed that natural killer activity was reduced in depressed people, but doubled after two weeks of treatment with an antidepressant, and returned to normal levels upon recovery.[20]

Other research has suggested that depressed people may be more susceptible to a reactivation of chicken pox, in the form of shingles, due to immune system suppression.[21] However, evidence to show that the immune system changes observed in the laboratory actually influence the risk of shingles in humans is still lacking.

The relationship between depression, immune system activity and infection is complex. Animals exposed to inescapable stress seem to adopt a behavioural state akin to depression (more of which later). There is compelling evidence that when in this state animals have an increased susceptibility to viral diseases such as herpes simplex and influenza, due to immune system malfunction.[22] However, because depression is often a *consequence* of chronic stress, it is hard to separate the effects of depression *per se* on immunity from the effects of chronic stress and anxiety that pre-date it. If we were to accept that depression is *not* synonymous with chronic stress, it would be hard to make the case that depression has an independent effect on infection risk. It seems that very stressed individuals are at a greater risk of infection, *regardless of whether or not they become depressed*. When a depression resolves, immune system function tends to return to normal, which is beneficial in the longer term. Furthermore, Michael Irwin, an expert in this area, has concluded that 'stress *and* depression can induce *increases as well as decreases* of immune function . . . depending on the immune measures and the chronicity [duration] of the stress' [my italics].[19]

Similar defences can be made when depression is accused of increasing the risk of most physical diseases, including heart disease, and of increasing mortality. Evidence has been presented which suggests that depression increases the risk of dying following a heart attack, for example.[23] Depression seems to predict mortality whether it is considered a disorder or an ongoing risk factor. This association with early death is not just limited to specific physical diseases – there is an increased risk in the mixed-disease populations of hospitals or nursing homes.[24,25] Complex models have been proposed which attempt to explain how depression can lead to disease. For example, the increased risk of heart disease in depressed patients is explained by depression's influence over increased blood pressure, variation in heart rate, increased platelet 'stickability', and increased immune system attack on our own artery walls.

However, all conclusions of the kind 'depression increases one's risk of developing disease', it 'speeds the progression of disease' or it 'increases disease severity' are beyond the data, and may be driven by a desire to medicalise the condition. Not only is there contradictory evidence, none of the research evidence can separate the effects of depression from the independent effects of the stress that pre-dated the depression, and which can impact on both physical and mental disease at the same time.

Furthermore, patients with depression generally have other risk factors for chronic disease. One has only to consider the association between depression and unemployment or poverty. Such social adversity can independently affect disease rates, not only through stress, but also through its association with poor diet, smoking, drinking and inactivity. Increasingly sophisticated studies of premature death have tried to control for these factors but apply to the elderly only and still have problems with method.[26]

Let us consider some of the contradictory evidence. Other studies have shown that there is no increased risk of death in depressed people with cancer or end-stage kidney disease.[27, 28,29] One study, published in the American Journal of Geriatric Psychiatry, concluded that the experience of subclinical depression had no effect on the lifespan of elderly men, and was associated with *reduced* mortality in elderly women.[30] Furthermore, a study attempting to show differences in heart rate variation in depressed individuals versus non depressed individuals following heart attack concluded that there was no difference.[31]

Although we know that depression is associated with immune and other internal physiological changes, a neat conclusion is provided by Michael Irwin: 'translation of these observations into clinical and disease-specific outcomes remains incomplete'.[19] So, with the current state of knowledge, a *causal* link between depression and physical disease cannot be made; there is merely an association. The 'depression-as-adaptation' idea is not under threat from the current evidence because one cannot conclude from it that depression causes disease.

Some important assumptions about depression

1 Depression is the product of nature and nurture, not one or the other. In most people it is triggered by stressful life events.
2 We all have the biological capacity for depression, to varying degrees. This is due to lots of genes, each of small effect, distributed over the whole population, acting together to cause susceptibility to depression. In other words, your genetic vulnerability depends on how many of these common genes (or types of gene variants) you have inherited from your parents. This is the lottery of meiosis following conception – the random jumbling of male and female deoxyribonucleic acid (DNA). The risk depends on how many relevant genes each of your parents are carrying, but you could be lucky and end up with very few. The picture is complicated because some common genes take more than one form, each carrying different risks for depression, and different genes may interact – they might act against each other or with each other. Hence, apart from inheriting more genes in total, you may inherit more potent versions of genes, or more genes that work together as a team to cause depression than your sibling. A good example of a gene that has forms of different potency is the 'serotonin transporter gene', which comes in short or long forms (s and l). It controls the turnover of the brain chemical serotonin, which is critical in the control of our moods. One large study, carried out on over 5000 children and young adults in Dunedin, New Zealand, demonstrated that, in those individuals who had experienced 4 or more adverse life events, their risk of depression was greatest in the s + s combination (an s inherited from both parents; occurring in 17% of the population), and smallest for l + l (an l from both parents; 30% of the population), with s + l falling in-between (s from one parent, l from the other).[32] The ss and sl forms make up 47% of the population.

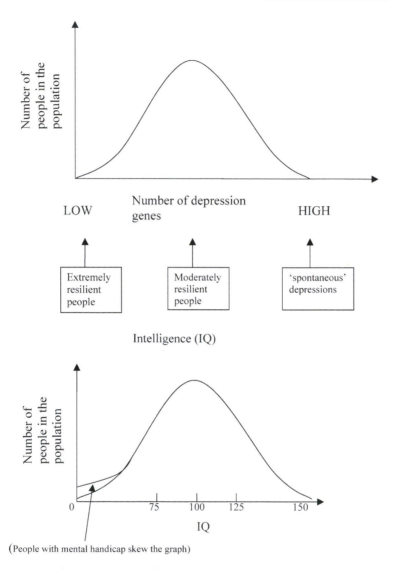

Figure 2 The genetic vulnerability to depression

3 However, the serotonin transporter gene is just one gene that is presumed to have an effect on depression. There will be many genes underlying our capacity for depression, each of small effect. I have assumed that genetic vulnerability is distributed across the

population like a bell curve, depending on the number and potency of genes inherited. The genes coding for IQ are a good analogy: most of us are of average intelligence but there will be a few geniuses and a few people who have significant learning difficulties. There is a tendency towards the mean. Similarly, I have assumed that most people will have *moderate* vulnerability to depression under stress; there will be a few people who have few or no depression genes and are highly resilient to stress; and there will also be rare individuals who have so many depression genes that they become depressed apparently 'spontaneously' – the so called 'endogenous depressives' (*see* Figure 2). The severity of depression that people experience is continuously variable, and I would expect that this is also under similar genetic control (when keeping the effects of the environment constant).

4 Psychological vulnerability – due to upbringing and adverse life experiences prior to the current crisis – acts in addition to the genetic vulnerability, and contributes to the risk of getting depressed in the face of stress occurring later on. The effects of upbringing and life difficulty explain why, in two identical twins, one can suffer depression and the other not (studies show that identical twins will both develop depression about 60% of the time, but that leaves 40% who do not). [33]

References

1 Tooby J and Cosmides L. The psychological foundations of culture. In Jerome H. Barkow, Leda Cosmides, and John Tooby, editors, *The adapted mind*, chapter 1, pages 19–136. Oxford University Press, Oxford, 1992.

2 Seligman MEP. Phobias and preparedness. *Behavior Therapy*, 1971; **2**: 307–320.

3 Garcia J and Koelling RA. Relation of cue to consequence in avoidance learning. *Psychonomic Science*, 1966; **4**: 123–4.

4 Buss DM. *Evolutionary Psychology: the new science of the mind*. London: Allyn and Bacon; 1999.

5 Resnik DB and Vorhaus DB. Genetic modification and genetic determinism.*Philos Ethics Humanit Med*. 2006; **1**(1): E9.

6 Gould SJ and Lewontin RC. The spandrels of San Marco and the Panglossian paradigm: a critique of the adaptationist programme. *Proceedings of the Royal Society of London. Series B, Containing papers of a Biological character.* 1979; **205**: 581–98.

7 Eaton SB, Cordain L and Lindeberg S. Evolutionary health promotion: a consideration of common counterarguments. *Preventive Medicine.* 2002; **34**: 109–18.

8 Darwin C. *The Origin of Species*, with introduction by *Julian Huxley*, Signet Classics 2003 edition.

9 Buist-Bouwman MA, Ormel J, de Graaf R and Vollebergh WAM. Functioning after a major depressive episode: complete or incomplete recovery? *Journal of Affective Disorders.* 2004; **82**: 363–71.

10 www.who.int/mental_health/prevention/suicide/suicideprevent/en/

11 Miles CP. Conditions predisposing to suicide: a review. *Journal of Nervous and Mental Disease.* 1977; **4**: 231–46.

12 World Health Organization. Depressive disorders in different cultures: Report of the WHO collaborative study of standardized assessment of depressive disorders. Geneva: WHO; 1983.

13 Chishti P, Stone DH, Corcoran P, Williamson E and Petridou E. EUROSAVE Working Group. Suicide mortality in the European Union. *Eur J Public Health.* 2003; **13**(2): 108–14.

14 Maris RW. Social and familial risk factors in suicidal behavior. *Psychiatr Clin North Am.* 1997; **20**(3): 519–50.

15 Coser and Lewis A. *Masters of Sociological Thought: Ideas in Historical and Social Context*, second edition. New York: Harcourt Brace Jovanovich; 1977.

16 The Evolution of Depression – Does it Have a Role? Broadcast on ABC Radio on Saturday 3 April 2004. Transcript available at www.abc.net.au/rn/science/buzz/

17 www.samaritans.org.uk

18 Jollant F, Bellivier F, Leboyer M, Astruc B, Torres S, Verdier R, Castelnau D, Malafosse A and Courtet P. Impaired decision making in suicide attempters. *Am J Psychiatry.* 2005; **162**(2): 304–10.

19 Irwin M. Presidential address. Psychoneuroimmunology of depression: clinical implications. *Brain, Behaviour and Immunity.* 2002; **16**: 1–16.

20 Kook AI, Mizruchin A, Odnopozov N, Gershon H and Segev Y. Depression and immunity: the biochemical interrelationship between the central nervous system and the immune system. *Biological Psychiatry.* 1995; **37**: 817–19.

21 Irwin M, Costlow C, Williams H Artin KH *et al.* Cellular immunity to varicella-zoster virus in depression. *Journal of Infectious Diseases.* 1998; **178**: S104–8.

22 Sheridan JF, Dobbs C, Brown D and Zwilling B. Psychoneuroimmunology: stress effects on pathogenesis and immunity during infection. *Clinical Microbiology Review.* 1994; **7**: 200–212.

23 Musselman DL, Evans DL and Nemeroff CB. The relationship of depression to cardiovascular disease: epidemiology, biology and treatment. *Archives of General Psychiatry.* 1998; **55;** 580–92.

24 Herrmann C, Brand-Driehorst S , Kaminsky B *et al.* Diagnostic groups and depressed mood as predictors of 22 month mortality in medical inpatients. *Psychosomatic Medicine.* 1998; **60**: 570–77.

25 Rovner BW. Depression and increased risk of mortality in the nursing home patient. *American Journal of Medicine.* 1993; **94**: 19S–22S.

26 Schulz R, Beach SR, Ives DG, Martire LM, Ariyo AA and Kop WJ. Association between depression and mortality in older adults: the Cardiovascular Health Study. *Archives of Internal Medicine.* 2000; **160**: 1761–68.

27 Christensen AJ, Wiebe JS, Smith TW and Turner CW. Predictors of survival among haemodialysis patients: effect of perceived life support. *Health Psychology.* 1994; **13**: 291–3.

28 Murphy KC, Jenkins PL and Whittaker JA. Psychosocial morbidity and survival in adult bone marrow transplant recipients – a follow-up study. *Bone Marrow Transplant.* 1996; **18**(1): 199–201.

29 Richardson JL, Zarnegar Z, Bisno B and Levine A. Psychosocial status at initiation of cancer treatment and survival. *Journal of Psychosomatic Research.* 1990; **34**: 189–201.

30 Hybels CF, Carl F, Pieper DPH and Blazer DG. Sex Differences in the Relationship Between Subthreshold Depression and Mortality in a Community Sample of Older Adults. *Am J Geriatr Psychiatry.* 2002; **10**: 283–291.

31 Gehi A, Mangano D, Pipkin S, Browner WS and Whooley MA. Depression and heart rate variability in patients with stable coronary heart disease: findings from the Heart and Soul Study. *Arch Gen Psychiatry.* 2005; **62**(6): 661–6.

32 Caspi A, Sugden K, Moffitt TE, Taylor A, Craig IW, Harrington H, McClay J, Mill J, Martin J, Braithwaite A and Poulton R. Related Articles, Links Influence of life stress on depression: moderation by a polymorphism in the 5-HTT gene. *Science.* 2003; **301**(5631): 386–9.

33 McGuffin P, Katz R, Watkins S and Rutherford J. A hospital-based twin register of the heritability of DSMIV unipolar depression. *Archives of General Psychiatry.* 1996; **53**: 129–136.

The war of depression: an ancient human condition or a modern malaise?

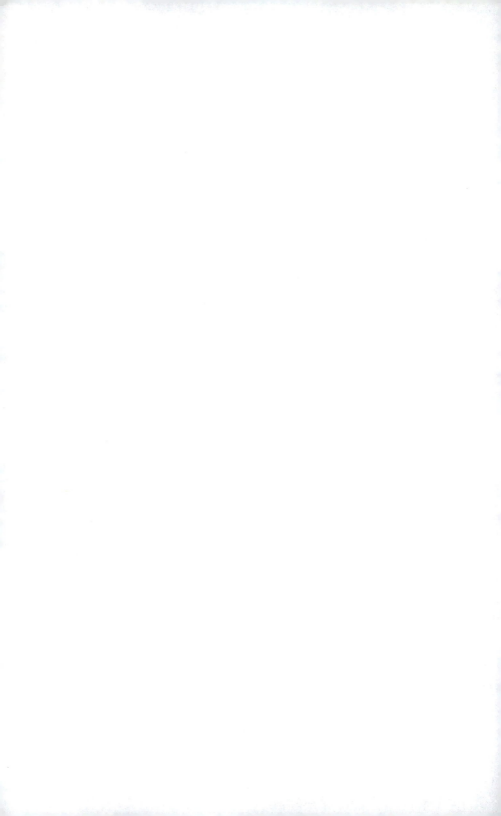

CHAPTER 1

Living on a boat

Marco lived on a yacht, moored at the ancient Spanish port of Vigo. Not a particularly impressive vessel, it was of modest proportions, but its decks were a clean white and its chrome gleamed. It contained all that he considered necessary to function comfortably from day to day – a fridge, stereo, cooker, shower. A moveable home, it could quickly put nautical miles between him and all the things that had made him depressed three years earlier in the big city.

When I was first introduced to Marco by my old friend Paula I had no idea that he had been depressed. It all came out, as is often the case, when he learned that I was a psychiatrist specialising in depression. It was now hard for most people to believe, he said, that he had once thought about ending his life. Marco had lived alone in a large apartment in the city, with a successful career designing sets for department stores and fashion shows. He was estranged from his family. Prior to his depression he had been caught up in a metropolitan whirl of parties and lunches. He had been a man with influential contacts, but he had also had a deep fear of being rejected, a barely hidden self-esteem problem, a highly stressful job, and a prodigious cocaine habit.

I did not pry into the details of Marco's past. It is possible that he was deprived of a warm and nurturing environment in his early years. All humans, and most higher mammals, need such an environment in order to maintain healthy relationships throughout life. If parental affection is lacking, a close attachment to at least one other significant adult will often suffice. Experience of emotional coldness in our early years can leave us with great difficulty forming lasting bonds with others as sexualised adults, often due to a persistent feeling of being unlovable and a fear of being abandoned.

The desire to be loved and the desire to belong are strong mammalian instincts. In fact, they define the mammal. Such instinctive needs are brought into even sharper focus by the segregating influences of modern urban society – mobile workforces, smaller families, jobless communities, and economic and social class.

We are archetypal social animals; our frontal lobes have developed and expanded in order to process and understand many different types of social behaviour. We excel at predicting the future behaviour of others, based on an accurate assessment of what their current behaviour reveals about their thoughts and feelings. How good we are at this is highlighted by the exceptions – people with conditions like autism – who seem to completely lack such fundamental capacities.

In short, we have become masters at empathy and at developing accurate theories about what others might be thinking, so that we can predict the needs and behaviours of others and hence minimise conflict. This has helped us to maintain social harmony within the tight-knit groups of the ancestral environment, ensure we get a share of resources, and avoid personal injury. A process of biological and cultural coevolution has occurred, by which I mean that individual humans have enjoyed a better chance of survival within groups, but that group rules have changed over time as a consequence of changes in biology. As our brains have become more sophisticated so have our cultures, and vice versa.

Material mechanisms in our brains influence our social calculations, or assessments of others, and also our own emotional reactions to these calculations. Whether these mechanisms are amenable to spiritual manipulation is open to endless debate, but such a debate is outside the realms of science. We cannot ignore biology, or the effect of natural selection, on emotional mechanisms.

The biology of our brains was shaped over a period of six million years, and for over 99.5 per cent of this time *Homo sapiens* lived in small groups of hunter–gatherers. Compared to this period of evolution the past few millennia or so of human civilisation – dating from the beginning of the Bronze Age – are a drop in the ocean. Advanced civilisation – the organisation of subject peoples within a large society, with armies and division of labour – has only been possible because of the relatively recent development of agriculture and animal husbandry. Biology takes a long time to catch up with changes in environment. Our brain mechanisms, although malleable and adaptable to cultural changes, have limits to their capability set by our ancestral heritage.

In the modern urban environment Marco's brain mechanisms were probably stretched to their limit and beyond. Cast adrift from family and friends, Marco chased material goals that were alien to the hunter–gatherer ancestors from whom we evolved. Marco lacked the frank feedback about his behaviour that he might have received in a more supportive community. He became trapped in interminable loops of worry and anxiety, ruminating about his place within a complex hierarchical system for which, arguably, his emotional mechanisms had not been designed.

We do better at surviving challenging new urban environments, from an emotional point of view, if we are securely attached to care-givers in our formative years – if our emotional knowledge tells us that we are complete, loveable, beings. But if we are unsure of ourselves, like Marco, the emotional and cognitive demands of modern city life can bring us to the brink of brain disorder: neural mechanisms and neurochemicals spiral into a new dimension, a new order, perhaps a state of psychiatric illness.

We may be witnessing an epidemic of insecurely attached, psychologically vulnerable individuals in modern urban society. As the extended family has been replaced by a smaller, more mobile one, balanced homes have been replaced by broken ones, rearing parents have become working ones, young parents have become more stressed and isolated; and we may have failed to rear our children effectively. Furthermore, we may have started to chase the wrong goals, or goals which are out of reach. We have exposed ourselves to ever-increasing work and social demands while turning our backs on mutual interdependence. In the west we have gained much more personal freedom and material wealth, but at a cost.

So, could it be that all common mental health problems, like depression, are just products of an environment that is at odds with our biology?

A good example of modern cultural pressures interacting with established brain mechanisms is anorexia nervosa. Anorexia nervosa is hardly ever found in the traditional tribes of rural Africa but it has become prevalent in capitalist western cultures where there are powerful media pressures to be thin, where dieting is commonplace, and where the need for personal control over eating is perceived as a priority. Modern pressures tap into formerly helpful mechanisms that enabled our ancestors to cope with periods of famine (i.e. the ability to suppress our hunger), but these mechanisms spiral out of control.[1]

Similarly, ischaemic heart disease (IHD) could represent a mismatch between recent cultural changes and ancient biology. IHD is extremely common in the developed world. The underlying disease process is a furring of the heart's arteries by a mixture of cholesterol and fat; it causes angina, or heart attack – the biggest killer in most western societies. The instincts of our ancestors to be attracted to the sweet and fatty foods that would have sustained them during the lean times, and the tendency of our bodies to store fat, lead to problems when nutritious food is readily available in the modern urban world, facilitated by recent developments in farming, agriculture, mass production and modern distribution systems. To compound the problem, our lives are generally more sedentary. We obtain food without having to work hard for it. Layers of fat are deposited in the artery walls of obese, immobile creatures.

Depression, it could be argued has arisen in the same way – due to a mismatch between evolved biology and culture. The lay view of depression is that it is a recent phenomenon, and one that is much more prevalent in the west. The logical progression of this modern malaise idea is that, in antiquity, when we existed in a presumably less complex, more harmonious and more natural environment, we would have been free of melancholy, just as a hunter–gatherer lifestyle and a more meagre diet would have made us immune to IHD and anorexia nervosa. This 'happy savage' notion has a long history in the European psychiatry movement, dating back to observations carried out by psychiatrists at the beginning of the twentieth century, who suggested that depression was relatively uncommon, or even absent, in the more traditional and isolated societies of the world. Some of these observers believed that the native brains were too primitive to experience such mood changes.

In addition to this there are recent observations by the WHO which show a rapid increase in depression rates worldwide.[2] The statistics cannot really be disputed. Depression is, apparently, a scourge of the new millennium, predicted to be second only to IHD as the leading cause of disability in the modern world by 2020. Could this be due to the spread of industrialised economies and the problems of urban living?

Also in support of the modern malaise idea are reports showing that the prevalence of depression in immigrant groups who have moved from traditional communities to cities of the modern western world is higher than in the culture of origin.[3] At face value this seems to provide support for the idea that depression is generated by urbanised living. An obvious challenge to this particular argument is that there are many other factors potentially operating in the environment of the immigrant, such as the experience of racism, or separation from loved ones in the country of origin, that independently affect depression. In any case, these findings do not imply that the prevalence of depression in the country of origin is zero.

The manifestation of all psychiatric conditions is probably affected by cultural change. This does not imply, however, that they spring from cultural pressures alone. The fact that depression is on the increase does not mean that it would have been absent in our ancestors.

There is increasing evidence to support the view that depression is not a modern malaise, but an ancient condition, and this will be presented in the next three chapters. Those readers who are already satisfied with the assertion that depression is universal, is inherited from other mammals, and has persisted since ancient times, can go straight to Section 3.

This is where I start to explore how depression could be an evolved mechanism for curtailing unhelpful thoughts and behaviours – an involuntary brake, which is activated when, for various reasons, we don't seem able to voluntarily give up on a futile and stressful quest. In other words I will explore the true *meaning* of depression; is it is telling us that we need to change the way we perceive ourselves or our situations?

I will examine why some people seem to carry on striving in spite of very little progress toward an ambition or goal, while neglecting their more pressing human needs, as determined by evolution (like the need to belong, or the need for a sexual relationship). There may be reasons that are to do with our situation; conflicts of interest, status battles, divided loyalties, threats to the survival of self and loved ones, or rejections and lost loves.[4] There may be internal reasons, to do with exaggerated expectations, low self-esteem, false information, lofty goals or high moral scruples, which keep us driving fruitlessly on, attempting perhaps to please everyone or achieve perfection in everything. These are timeless dilemmas, but they are made worse by features of the modern developed world like the media.

Depression, it has been suggested, is triggered in situations of failing to achieve a goal. It may have evolved to put a check on people whose aspirations exceed their abilities, and it may remind them of their true place in any hierarchy. The idea that depression is all about loss of rank and status has been around since the late 1960s, but is far from mainstream.

I will argue that this theory has some merit but is incomplete. In my view the overriding meaning behind depression is the frustration of 'archetypal needs', over a protracted period of time, because of fighting to achieve abstract goals. In other words, the status goal or the strategy for achieving it is often wrong – we need to change the goal or be more patient in achieving it. Our goals should lead to a satisfaction of archetypal needs, rather than hinder them; otherwise they are not suitable goals at all.

Archetypal needs are instinctive and unconscious. They do not need to be learnt. They have a bearing on our differential reproductive success and our survival: they include the need for shelter and security, the need for sustenance, the need for parental nurturing, the need for a loving partnership, the need for inclusion in a group, and the need for status in a group. We do not become depressed if an obstacle to these goals arises only briefly – in fact, we tend to try harder (the feeling of being stressed drives us to do this), or we find a different strategy, and this usually pays off. However, more persistent obstacles, either internal or external, cause long-term stress. This *protracted* stress can, and probably will, lead to depression. So, depression is caused by *protracted frustration of archetypal* needs. In the fast pace of urban living we frequently forget what our archetypal needs are. For optimum happiness we need to fulfil each one, and in the right order of priority. This means gaining a deeper understanding of the self, one that can only come about through prolonged introspection.

So, like sadness, depression may serve an essential *reassessment* function. The reassessment is facilitated by sad mood, which pares away the excessively optimistic, illusional thinking of the non-depressed person, leaving only stark reality. This leads to enlightenment and a change in behaviour in the future. In the case of ordinary sadness, perhaps consequent upon losing a 100 m athletic event, or failing an exam, the solution becomes apparent quickly and relatively painlessly. We might resolve, over the coming days, to train harder, compete in a different event or a different sport, study harder, or find solace in other achievements. However, the changes in behaviour required after the onset of depression, in order to prevent further depressions, are likely to be more fundamental or more *radical* than the remedies required after merely losing a race, or failing an exam. For example, Marco's decision to make a yacht his home was a truly radical one, which arose from deeper and longer-lasting problems.

Marco believed that everyone should go through depression in order to discover who they really were, what their fundamental needs were, and how to go about meeting them effectively, and that only *in extremis* could we do this. For him, depression was part of growing up, of reaching full maturity – a thirty-something rite of passage which had led to greater inner peace. He could stand back and observe his old friends, many of them displaying signs of what he regarded as a desperate desire to be loved and accepted, still exposed to the most destructive aspects of city life, struggling on in quiet desperation, trying to be top of the pile, while at the same time trying to please everyone in spite of themselves.

He concluded, not without irony, that some people would never be content unless they first of all became depressed. He believed that, although depression was an incredibly painful experience, it could ultimately liberate people from their emotional disabilities and innermost fears.

The evolutionary perspective has far-reaching implications for the treatment and prevention of depression. For example, if mild-to-moderate depression is so helpful, why should we treat it? These issues will be explored in the final part of the book. First of all we will consider the history of depression.

References

1   Stevens A, Price J. *Evolutionary psychiatry: a new beginning.* London: Routledge; 2000.

2   World Health Organization. *World health report: conquering suffering, enriching humanity.* Geneva: World Health Organization; 1997.

3   Vega W, Rumbaut R. Ethnic minorities and mental health. *Annual Review of Sociology.* 1991; **7**: 351–83.

4   Price J. The adaptive function of mood change. *British Journal of Medical Psychology.*1998; **71**: 465–77.

CHAPTER 2

Why weepest thou?

Most books that have been written on the history of psychiatry do not go back further than the last two centuries. Ignorance of history can lead us to the often misguided view that society's current problems are new. It follows that if we have no knowledge of depression occurring in ancient times it is tempting to believe that it is a creation of modern life. We have only recently started to look for accounts of depression in ancient texts, so challenging the idea that depression is a modern malaise is quite new.

For example, there appears to be evidence of depression in the Bible. The Old Testament was written between 2000 and 3000 years ago. In the beginning of the Book of Samuel, Elkannah asks of his wife 'Why weepest thou? Why eatest thou not? And why is thy heart grieved?' (Samuel 1:8). Also, consider the Book of Job. Job lived in the fourth century before Christ. He is thought to have been a prosperous nomad, living in south-east Palestine. According to the biblical story he loses all of his children 'to Satan' and suffers from a severe skin condition, which some physicians suggest might have been psychosomatic. Job provides a vivid description of the depressed state:

20 Why is light given to those in misery,
and life to the bitter of soul,
21 to those who long for death that does not come,
who search for it more than for hidden treasure,
22 who are filled with gladness
and rejoice when they reach the grave?
23 Why is life given to a man
whose way is hidden,
whom God has hedged in?
24 For sighing comes to me instead of food;
my groans pour out like water.
25 What I feared has come upon me;

what I dreaded has happened to me.
26 I have no peace, no quietness;
I have no rest, but only turmoil. (Job 3: 20–26)
. . .

3 so I have been allotted months of futility,
and nights of misery have been assigned to me.
4 When I lie down I think, 'How long before I get up?'
The night drags on, and I toss till dawn.
5 My body is clothed with worms and scabs,
my skin is broken and festering.
6 My days are swifter than a weaver's shuttle,
and they come to an end without hope. (Job 7: 3–6)

Although Job contemplates death, he never refers to suicide, but rather considers how he can transcend his despair: 'I am not silenced by the darkness, by the thick darkness that covers my face.' (Job 23: 17). For some sufferers of depression Job's strength has provided solace and encouragement. For example, Soren Kierkegaard (1813–1855) wrote:

Every word of Job is nourishment and clothing and medicine for the misery of the soul. At times a word of his arouses me from my lethargy, so that I wake up to a new restlessness, at times it silences the fruitless rage inside myself, ends the horror in a silent rattle of passion.[1]

The ancient Greeks were the first writers to coin the phrase 'melancholia', literally meaning 'black bile'.[2] Celsus, a physician to the Roman Army, and the attending doctor during many gladiatorial battles, was a major proponent of the concept of 'black bile disease', which he said manifested itself in 'prolonged sadness and sleeplessness and fearfulness'. He noted that such melancholy could sometimes be relieved by 'soft music', but he also advocated the much harsher treatment of induced vomiting for 'melancholy without fever', reflecting an obsession with the ejection of foul bile from the circulation.

Not all the Greeks believed in the black bile theory. Hippocrates stated that 'from the brain, and from the brain only, arise our pleasures, joys . . . as well as our sorrows, pain, grief and tears'. As an ancient precursor of modern pharmaceutical remedies for depression, he advocated treating melancholy with the drug hellebore, which was prepared from the white lily. The Greek physician Galen was also more concerned with the brain than the circulation. He believed that the soul was located in the 'nerve centres', and that the brain was the centre of all psychic functions.

Ancient Indian texts also reveal knowledge of a state akin to depression. The *Rig Veda*, thought to be the world's oldest book, describes the state known as the *manes*.[3] The *manes* was attributed to malign spiritual forces, as invisible as the sun's rays. It was characterised by agitated looks, somnolence, impaired speech, apathy with regard to eating food, anorexia, and indigestion. Ayurvedic texts, and several Vedic hymns, contain vivid descriptions of a state that can only be conceptualised as depression: 'Sufferers are mute, rooted to one spot and dribbling saliva, with loss of appetite, somnolence, self-neglect, pale white face [possibly due to withdrawing from social contact and staying indoors], fixed eyes, glazed look and preference for solitude.' The 'obedient and obliging' personality that is said to predispose to this condition is similar to the 'depressive position' described by some modern psychoanalysts, after Melanie Klein, and modern concepts of low self-esteem, which is thought to predispose to depression.[4]

In the *Ramayana*, Lord Rama appears to become depressed.[5] He loses weight through his protracted mental torment, his 'once radiant body' becoming 'all at once emaciated like the river floods subsiding in the summer'. His red face becomes wan, his mood despondent. He becomes 'absorbed in pensive thought', forgetting to perform his 'allotted duties of life'. His guru notes that Rama's condition is far more severe than any ordinary reaction to the loss of a desired object, or any disappointment arising out of 'great accident.'

Rama's condition was clearly not a transient one. It must have persisted for weeks in order to cause such a change in his weight and appearance. Also, his elder relatives developed similar mental states, suggesting that depressive-like states were known to run in families, just as we observe now. Lord Rama's grandfather starved himself to death after his wife's death, and Rama's father suffered from three melancholy-like episodes, each following some terrible life event – his accidental killing of a blind man, and two enforced separations from his children. In keeping with the fates of his father and his son, and for the purposes of tragic drama, the last of these melancholic episodes results in death.

The *Mahabharata* describes an early form of psychotherapy for depression, in the form of counselling provided by Lord Krishna, which brings about speedy relief of the depressive-type symptoms in our protagonist, Arjun.[6] In the *Ayurveda*, psychotherapy for any 'mental imbalance' is prescribed according to the type of excessive emotion.[3] It is said that any excess of grief should be allayed by bringing the influence of opposite emotions to bear on the prevailing mood in order to neutralise it.

It was also Ayurvedic practice to treat someone who had a 'mental imbalance due to loss', by offering 'a substitute or, if it be not possible, words of sympathy and comfort'. Massage with oils, lying in the sun, and being kept in comfortable rooms without draughts, were other methods employed to manage depression-like states.

Melancholy was by far the most important disorder among the Incas of ancient Peru to be documented by the Spanish chroniclers at the time of the conquests.[7] The third principal wife of the first Inca ruler was 'very depressive', 'wept about insignificant matters', and 'ate little or nothing', instead consuming 'a lot of chicha', which was the alcoholic drink of the Incas, and was also a treatment for depressive states. The fourth Inca ruler is described as a melancholic man, and the wife of the eighth Inca ruler is described as 'very melancholic, weeping for insignificant things, and feeling wretched'. Melancholy was relatively common, it seems, among the Inca ruling elite, and there is a suggestion once again of the condition tending to 'run in the family'.

The large number of plants used to treat melancholy following the Spanish conquest of Peru suggests that the condition was common and widespread. Fifteen different plants were used for this purpose – nearly as many as the number of different antidepressants in common use today. Some of these may have been brought across by the Spanish. They included euphorbia, cassia and china root. The seeds of the *guayroro* and *vilca* were ground for consumption with water, or in the alcoholic drink *chicha*. Preparations from the flowers (extract of pupa flower) and leaves (decoctions of *hampeani, mocomoco, mutoy, yuralmayacha* and *harachigua* leaves) were used. Some plant preparations were used in magical ways. For example, the *guayroro* beans were worn as a necklace around the neck to cure depression. Also, the powder of the *siasa* tree was thought to cure depression when applied over the heart.

A number of minerals, including the *piedra lipez*, and *piedra lazuli*, were also used to treat melancholia. Some were taken together with bezoar stone (a conglomerate formed by hairballs in animal stomachs, as this was thought to enhance the action of the mineral. The bezoar stone and the *piedro lipez* were common European remedies, and were probably brought to South America by the Spanish. The *coco de Paraguay*, thus named because of the place where it was first discovered by the colonists, was also a highly prized treatment for depression.

We know from contemporary Peruvian communities that a form of psychotherapy has long been an important treatment for depression, and it is still practised today by indigenous shamans or *curenderos*. It is highly likely that these talking therapies are ancient traditions, but the Spanish chroniclers had little interest in them, being more concerned with the medicinal preparations that could be added to their pharmacopeia back in Spain.

One must bear in mind, when interpreting the Spanish chronicles, that they were often written a considerable time after the conquest, that the chroniclers only recorded what they considered to be important, and that they often had relatively little experience with medical matters. For these reasons it is difficult to make definitive statements about the prevalence of depressive illness in the ancient Inca societies, although we can be fairly confident that depressive illness, in the contemporary sense, existed then.

Meanwhile, Burton, a scholar and diviner, came to Oxford University in 1593 to devote himself to his classic work *The Anatomy of Melancholy*.[8] This was published in 1621, when he was 44, the result of a life's dedication to the furtherance of an understanding of mental illness 'philosophically, medically, and historically'. He did not use the term melancholy in this context in the same sense in which it was used by the Greeks or the Spanish chroniclers. It was a catch-all term for a state halfway between madness and folly, and was often used figuratively as a way of expressing the stupidity of mankind, as to Burton the world seemed deranged, a 'vast confusion of vows, wishes, actions, law-suits, laws, complaints and proclamations'. Burton believed that self-knowledge would lead man to conduct himself more wisely.

However, although he was a philosopher, Burton was also concerned with 'anatomising', or analysing, different types of behaviour that he regarded as irrational. In other words, he was also engaged in observing different types of mental illness and making studious attempts to delineate them. He identified one condition that he called 'sad melancholy'.

Burton's descriptions of sad melancholy could only have made reference to an illness that we would now call depression. The sadness of sad melancholy was 'haunting and continuous':

Like a vulture, it continuously gnawed at the melancholic man, and though, on some occasions, he might appear to have escaped it, to laugh and smile in congenial company, sorrow hovered over him like a bird of prey. He, the melancholic, was always sighing, pining, fretting, and weeping.

His concept of sad melancholy was summed up in a poem, his own composition, which features at the beginning of his book:

When I lie waking all alone,
Recounting what I have ill done,
My thoughts on me then tyrannise,
Feare and sorrow me surprise,
Whether I tarry still or goe,
Me thinkes the time moves very sloe.
All my griefes to this are jolly,
Naught so sad as Melancholy.

In sad melancholy there were 'signs of the minde' and 'signs of the body'. In examining these 'signs of the minde', he noted that the sad melancholic would tend to:

worry himself unnecessarily over other people's affairs and discontents; and about a past he could neither change nor affect. Digging up the dead memories of old affairs, disgraces, losses or injuries, he would begin worrying afresh about his past discontents, thus driving himself to perpetual agony.

Contemporary psychiatrists like Aaron T Beck have shown that depressed people tend towards a negative bias when appraising their pasts, having a selective memory for failures over successes.[9,10]

Burton was aware of the risk of suicide in the melancholic person. He noted that if someone's melancholia were to progress to a 'desperate and damned' state, he would consider himself the lowest of the low, deduce that his life is pointless, and conclude that it should be brought to an end. Thus, melancholia could drive a person to 'hange himself off cross-beams', 'drown [himself] in a poole', or 'praecipitate himselfe of a steep hill'. The twelfth stanza of his poem describes the melancholic who is close to suicide:

Ile change my state with any wretch,
Thou canst from geale or dunghill fetch:
My paines past cure, another Hell,
I may not in this torment dwell,
Now desperate I hate my life,
Lend me an halter or a knife.
All my griefes to this are jolly,
Naught so damn'd as melancholy.[8]

The signs of the body that Burton attributed to melancholy are the same as those we observe today. They include weight loss, manifested in the 'lean, withered, hollow-eyed man', abnormal bowel movements, 'little or no sleepe', and various symptoms of associated anxiety: 'singing in the ears, vertigo, light-headedness, cold sweats or even palpitations of the heart'.

Not surprisingly, during the time of the Spanish inquisition, the proposed causes for melancholy included demonic possession. However, more interestingly, the ordinary man's melancholy could be brought on by fear, sorrow, shame, disgrace, envy, malice, hatred, anger, discontent, 'cares' and 'miseries'.

Melancholy could be caused by such 'passions and perturbations', but could equally be cured, it was thought, by purging oneself of the passions that triggered it. Even more interestingly, Burton stressed the importance of a gaining of 'self-knowledge' to understand how these passions could have arisen, and thus find a way out of one's melancholia, and build strength for the future. These ideas could have been the seeds of a psychotherapeutic movement, but Burton himself advocated distraction from unhelpful thoughts, by substituting more pleasant or irrelevant thoughts, or purging them by confessing one's thoughts and feelings to a friend.

The recording of events in text, and the subsequent interpretation of this text, can never be purely objective. However, even accounting for interpretation, there is a persuasive body of evidence which suggests that depression dates back to the limits of history.

However, depression could still be a result of fairly recent advances in civilisation. We cannot discount the notion that depression was absent *before* recorded history using arguments based on historical evidence alone. The time span of recorded history is merely a drop in the ocean of human evolution – a process that has taken millions of years, and which has always occurred at a slow pace. For most of that time we have not been 'civilised'. We need to look for other evidence to determine just how ancient depression might be. One method is to examine the more traditional communities of today, to look for evidence of depression's universality across 'undeveloped' and 'developed' cultures.

References

1 Van Lieburg MJ. *Famous depressives: ten historical sketches*. Champagne Illinois: Erasmus Publishing; 1988.

2 Stone MH. *Healing the mind: a history of psychiatry from antiquity to the present*. New York: Norton; 1997.

3 Bhugra D. Psychiatry in ancient Indian texts: a review. *History of Psychiatry*. 1992; **3**: 167–86.

4 Hinshelwood R, Robinson S, Zarate O. *Introducing Melanie Klein*. Cambridge: Icon Books; 2005.

5 *Narayan RK. The Ramayana*. London: Penguin; 1977.

6 *Narayan RK. The Mahabharata*. London: Penguin; 2001.

7 Elferink JGR. Mental disorder among the Incas in ancient Peru. *History of Psychiatry*. 1999; **10**: 303–18.

8 Cox-Maksimov DCT. Burton's anatomy of melancholy: philosophically, medically and historically: part 2. *History of Psychiatry*. 1996; **7**: 343–59.

9 Beck, AT. *Cognitive therapy and the emotional disorders*. 4th ed. Madison, CT: International University Press Inc.; 1976.

10 Beck, AT, Rush, A J, Shaw, BF *et al. Cognitive therapy of depression*. New York: Guilford; 1979.

CHAPTER 3

Is depression universal?

Charles Darwin, who was himself prone to depression, published *The Expression of the Emotions in Animals and Man* in 1872, 13 years after *Origin of Species*.[1,2] This was the first large-scale attempt by a scientist to demonstrate that certain universals might exist in human emotional expression. Darwin wanted to support his theory of evolution – that we had all evolved from a common progenitor – by showing not only that certain emotional expressions were universal, and therefore had a common genetic blueprint, but also that there was some continuity between humans and other mammals in the way that we expressed moods. Some photographs of his observed expressions are shown in Figure 3.1.

Darwin interviewed people who had lived or travelled in foreign lands. He pointed to similarities in emotional expression across different cultures. He also recounted striking and poignant descriptions of grief or sadness in other mammals. On Indian elephants, captured in Ceylon (now Malaysia), he quoted an observer: '[the elephants] lay motionless on the ground, with no other indication of suffering than the tears which suffused their eyes and flowed incessantly'.[1]

Darwin's volume persuasively suggested that the influence of natural selection is not limited to mere physical characteristics but shapes our emotions. However, ever since its publication violent battles have been waged over the interpretation of its findings. Among the main players in this drama during the twentieth century have been the famous anthropologist Margaret Mead and, later, the experimental psychologist Paul Ekman.

Margaret Mead conducted detailed observations of many relatively isolated cultures. Her descriptions demonstrated that there were huge variations in behaviour – how people lived, hunted, fed, worked, formed intimate partnerships and raised their children – across the different cultures. In 1935 Margaret Mead published an academic work called *Sex and Temperament in Three Societies*, in which she

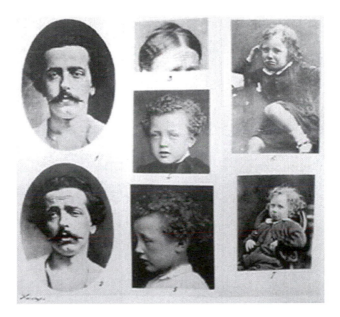

Figure 3.1   A picture taken from Darwin's book *The Expression of the Emotions in Animals and Man and Animals* demonstrating sadness

concluded that 'human nature is almost unbelievably malleable, responding accurately and contrastingly to contrasting cultural conditions.'[3] This 'cultural relativism' was, at the time, a welcome backlash against racism and eugenics, and it arose in the climate of radical behaviourism, which suggested that we are all entirely products of learning and experience.

This arguably optimistic stance suggested that individual differences could be wiped out if we were all raised in the same environment and with limitless opportunities for self-improvement. It further suggested that there were no genetic limits to our achievements. With regard to our emotional worlds, emotional displays were determined entirely by learnt rules of communication within a culture. There was no contribution from biology. It followed that some expressions, like a frown, could represent happiness in one culture, and displeasure in another; and that some facial expressions could be found in one culture and not in another. The cultural relativists would have strongly resisted any suggestion that the same symptoms of depression could be detected in every culture of the world. This would have implied a universal genetic liability, and even continuity with the animal kingdom.

Unfortunately for Margaret Mead, at the time that she was writing other researchers, most notably the developmental psychologist Florence Goodenough, were coming up with sound evidence to support Darwin's belief in emotional universality. More importantly, they provided direct support for the idea that emotional expressions were innate, not learned. They observed the emotional reactions of children who had not had the opportunity to imitate the emotional expressions of others. In 1932 Goodenough published her observations of a ten-year-old girl who had been blind and deaf from birth.[4] According to Goodenough, this young girl showed surprise when something unexpected happened, displayed sadness when a favourite toy was taken from her, and laughed and smiled when fun or pleasant objects were given to her. (In fact, prior to Goodenough's seminal paper, Darwin had observed that blind children seemed to 'blush with shame' and show other expressions in a manner similar to sighted children.[1]) Goodenough concluded that children who are born deaf and blind use the same facial expressions as other children to express the same emotions.

Goodenough blazed a trail for other researchers like Jane Thompson and Irenäus Eibl-Eibesfeldt, a German ethologist. Thompson took photographs of the emotional reactions of 26 blind children, aged from seven weeks to thirteen years, to certain situations, and had independent raters compare these reactions to those of sighted children, matched for age in similar emotion-provoking situations.[5] In the 1960s Eibl-Eibesfeldt went further and explored the role of IQ in a small number of children affected by thalidomide.[6] (Thalidomide was a drug, launched in the 1960s, which was found to cause major congenital defects to the unborn babies of pregnant women who took the drug, including eye, ear and brain defects.) The children in Eibl-Eibesfeldt's study were all deaf and blind from birth and had varying amounts of brain damage. They also had limb malformations. He videotaped the young children and then slowly played the tapes back. He observed a wide spectrum of spontaneous emotional expressions in each child, including smiling, crying, surprise, and frowning, which were similar to expressions shown by sighted children. This was true even of one child with an IQ within the severely disabled range. Other researchers produced similar results.[7,8]

Of course, all these studies had some weaknesses of method, but taken together they seem to imply that no social learning of emotional expression is required. This seems to be in direct contradiction to the findings of Margaret Mead, who had carefully observed differences in emotion expression across cultures.[3] Both theories could not be right as absolutes.

However, the most useful theory of human emotional expression came along later, in the 1970s. This theory, developed by the eminent experimental psychologist Paul Ekman, inhabited the middle ground.[9] Ekman used culture-sensitive observation techniques to demonstrate that the basic expressions of sadness, fear, disgust, anger and surprise could be found in many different cultures of the world, if one only took care to separate the *innate* behaviour from the *learned*. In other words, he showed that all cultures had the fundamental capacity to instinctively express these emotions in the same way, but that certain culture-specific display rules affected *when* they would be expressed.

For example, in the 1970s Ekman challenged the prevailing view that the Japanese did not express emotions in the same way as Americans. He did this by asking both Japanese and American people to watch an emotive film on two occasions – once in the presence of a 'scientist', dressed in a white coat, and once on their own. On both occasions their external expressions were recorded with a hidden camera. During the viewings with the 'scientist' present the Japanese did not express emotion as much as the Americans. However, when both Japanese and American people viewed the same film *on their own* they reacted in *very similar ways*. The suppression of emotional expression witnessed in the Japanese when the 'scientist' was present reflected a learned response to the presence of authority figures, defined by the Japanese culture. Without knowledge of this Japanese display rule one might have concluded, on the basis of crude observation, that the Japanese did not have the same innate range of emotional expressions as the Americans. This would have been a mistake.

These issues demonstrate the difficulties that can be anticipated in trying to detect a common collection of depressive symptoms in many different cultures. We are not merely considering the outward expressions of sadness, or lack of animation, we must also gain access to the inner thoughts and feelings, the communication of which is surely even more amenable to cultural variation. The cultural relativists, like Margaret Mead, would argue that it is impossible to find core features of depression that are present in all cultures of the world because there are more differences in the way that people express mental distress between cultures than there are similarities.[3] They would suggest that the presentation of mental distress in each culture is unique. It would be meaningless to look for universal features of depression across cultures if a person's psychiatric symptoms were entirely determined by the relationship he had with his society.

Differences exist, for example, in the physical location of sadness in different cultures – some feel sadness in the heart (the western concept), others in the stomach (like the Japanese). If Europe, which is the parent of modern psychiatry, devises a test for depression, it will use for its template the symptoms suffered by depressed people in Europe. Exaggerated guilt, which is unreasonable in context, is a common feature of depression in European and American cultures. However, it may be a rare feature of depression in India. Guilt may be particularly western. Many reasons for this have been postulated, including the contribution of the work ethic, and, in the older generation, the need to ration one's desires during the two World Wars. There may have been religious contributions too – from Lutheran Protestant and Catholic confessional traditions.

It is possible, however, that while some symptoms may be culture-bound, and so will be missed entirely in some cultures, other core symptoms may be universal. The development of the WHO's Standardised Assessment of Depressive Disorders (SADD) was the first large-scale attempt at producing a culturally unbiased interview for the diagnosis of depression.[10] It was used in the psychiatric populations of Basle, Montreal, Nagasaki, Teheran and Tokyo and was conducted by people from the host culture. Evidence could be gleaned from the local psychiatrist who had been treating the patient.

It was discovered that there were certain core symptoms of depression that were present in all cultures, and in at least 79 per cent of the total sample of patients. These symptoms included sadness, joylessness, hopelessness, anxiety, tension, lack of energy loss of interest, poor concentration, and feelings of insufficiency, inadequacy and worthlessness. The WHO study confirmed that excessive, often delusional, feelings of guilt or impoverishment and low self-esteem were particularly western expressions of depression. Delusions of guilt were completely absent in Teheran, and delusions of impoverishment absent in Tokyo.

Therefore, there were certain *core* symptoms of depression, sufficient for making a reliable diagnosis, present in all cultures studied. In addition, there were culturally specific symptoms, but these were less important than the universal ones.

The WHO study could be criticised for focusing on urban populations only. Its conclusions would not necessarily apply to a traditional African agricultural village. However, other studies have added to our knowledge of universal symptoms. Patients defined as depressed by local psychiatrists in Ghana had the same pattern of core symptoms, in roughly the same proportion (76 per cent or more of patients).[11] In China, a western psychiatrist called Kleinman found that the main core symptoms of depression were present in 87 per cent of patients presenting to Chinese psychiatrists with neurasthenia (or nervous exhaustion).[12] The label was different but the phenomenon was just the same, and many improved when given antidepressants.

The WHO study could also be criticised for using preconceived notions of how symptoms might aggregate together to form the depressive syndrome. An anthropologist called Morton Beiser and his colleagues attempted to show how similar psychological symptoms might occur frequently together in different cultures *without using any preconceived European notion of the nature of depressive symptoms.*[13] The aim was to see which generic symptoms of psychological distress tended to group together most often in different parts of the world. It was only later that these groupings were compared with our western concepts of diagnostic syndromes, including depression.

Beiser *et al.* studied the Serer, a community of settled agriculturalists who have inhabited Senegal for at least the past seven hundred years. They focused on the region of Niakur, where, at the time of the survey in 1970, the 35,000 inhabitants lived one of the most traditional lifestyles in Senegal, or possibly in the whole of West Africa. Four-hundred and forty-six adults, who were indigenously defined as probable psychiatric cases, were interviewed in their local tongue, Serer, about their distress. Over 100 different symptoms were described by this community, and they were compared with symptoms volunteered by communities in the Brooklyn and Queens suburbs of New York, and by a community of refugees from Vietnam, Laos and Cambodia who had resettled in Vancouver, British Columbia, during 1979 and 1980.

The over 100 items were a 'distillation of decades, if not centuries, of clinical lore' about the ways people report distress. All three communities were rated on all the symptoms, although symptoms that recorded a less than 10 per cent positive response across all three centres were excluded. No predetermined ideas were formed about which of these psychological symptoms might constitute the syndrome of depression. Instead, the researchers determined which symptoms seemed to occur most frequently together in each affected person, using a statistical technique called factor analysis.

The ingenuity of the design enabled the researchers to explore a wide range of psychological and psychosomatic symptoms, including items that had originally been regarded as culture specific.

The factor analysis revealed many clusters of symptoms, and one of these clusters contained the constellation of symptoms that western psychiatry would use to define depression.

In all centres, a significant proportion of all the symptoms reported were psychic descriptions of the depressive experience. The six symptoms presenting in all three cultures were hopelessness, indecisiveness, feelings of futility, hypersensitivity to the feelings of others, and anergia (lack of energy). Another group, called 'somatisation' (that is, describing distress in physical terms), could be separated out from these symptoms. The 'somatisation factor' included complaints about shortness of breath, palpitations, dizziness and persistent poor health. The 'depression dimension' was independent of scores on the somatisation dimension.

This latter finding was thought to be important because it challenged the prevailing view that non-western communities were unable to express depression in psychic terms, tending to perceive their distress in physical terms.

The WHO and Beiser *et al.* surveys challenge the extreme social–anthropological view that mental distress expresses itself in such radically different forms in different cultures as to make meaningless transcultural comparisons of the prevalence of a concept such as depression.[10,13] If depression has many core features that are evident across different continents it becomes meaningful to compare the prevalence of depression across cultures.

We know that major depression is common in the western world. However, for many decades, psychiatrists from the white western Christian culture such as Frederick Kraupl-Taylor, a professor of psychiatry during the first half of the twentieth century, have believed that the prevalence of depression in the 'undeveloped' cultures of Asia, Africa and South America is much lower than the western prevalence.[14] Some have even concluded that depression is non-existent in the traditional, 'undeveloped' communities.

These early researchers have mostly attributed this discrepancy to 'cultural differences'. Some, like Kraupl-Taylor, blamed the discrepancy on the less developed use of language in pre-literate societies. However, the most predominant explanation was that there were fewer stresses in the seemingly less complicated lives of the tribes of, say, traditional Africa, or Papua New Guinea. Carrothers, in his 1953 monograph *The African Mind in Health and Disease*, concluded that Africans did not suffer depression because of the 'lack of responsibility' they enjoyed within a 'primitive paradise'.[15]

This 'happy savage' idea persists to this day, despite the fact that people all over the world have had to deal with personal and interpersonal difficulties and tragedies – death of loved ones, separation from loved ones, status battles, childcare, ill-health and old age. As social animals we all have the potential to hurt each other, psychologically and emotionally, wherever we live, and extraneous stressors, acts of God and so on, can never be ruled out. In the modern world these stressors might be redundancy and crime; our ancestors would have had to endure famine and drought.

Some psychiatrists have suggested that the minds of the members of traditional communities are more primitive, and that this makes them less susceptible to depression. Kraepelin visited Java at the beginning of the twentieth century and concluded that depression was seldom experienced there.[16] He believed that the Indonesians were incapable of experiencing such a condition because they lacked the mental capacity to experience it. The underlying assumption was that their brains were less developed than the modern European brain – and consequently they had not evolved the capacity to experience depressed mood to the same degree. Forty years later, when biological explanations for mental illness and physical treatments such as lobotomy (making lesions in the frontal lobes of the brain) were all the rage, some psychiatrists even ventured to suggest that the African tribesman had an emotional life akin to the lobotomised European patient.

Early observations by European researchers in Africa and India often supported such beliefs by reporting low hospital admission rates for depression compared to Europe. For example Shaw, in his book entitled *Clinical Handbook of Mental Diseases* (published in 1925), reported that Indians in the Berhampore asylum suffered less frequently from depression than in-patients in European asylums.[17]

However, there were many reasons for these comparatively low estimates that had nothing to do with the true prevalence in the communities observed. First, little consideration was given to the possibility that many people with depression were not being admitted to hospital. This was indeed the case in many instances due to the very real barriers to hospital admission. Hospitals were often geographically remote, there was frequently a shortage of beds and there were limited primary care facilities for referral of patients to hospital.

Second, few depressed people attended local doctors, preferring instead to visit religious healers. Spiritual explanations for depression are common around the world. Such explanations can prevent people with the illness from coming forward for treatment. In India, the suffering that occurs during a depressive illness is often thought to be a punishment for sins in a past life. The self-prescribed treatment is to cry silently, work hard and pray. People living in India are willing to go to their doctor with physical complaints, but prefer to visit a spiritual healer for help with the mental distress caused by depression. Sudhir Kakar, a psychoanalyst working in India, conducted an anthropological study of the various ways in which mental health problems are treated there.[18] He identified three main kinds of care – the exorcism tradition, the Ayurvedic tradition and the Guru tradition. In the exorcism tradition there is a hierarchy of treatment: from the healer in the village up to the priest in the temple. The more intractable problems are treated in the temple. In the Ayurvedic tradition, treatments include herbs with tranquillising properties or shock treatment – using irritants placed up the nose, for example. The Guru tradition was the mainstay of treatment for depression.

So, in order to obtain an estimate of the true prevalence of depression in different countries, attempts have been made to conduct community surveys. Surveys can be fraught with difficulties.

One major difficulty is observer bias. Some early researchers, who, due to various preconceived notions (perhaps with their roots in the happy savage idea), were expecting low rates of depression, were not exactly painstaking in their attempts to detect the condition. Similar mistakes continue to be made in assessing contemporary immigrant communities in the western world. While I was a non-tenured researcher for BBC Radio Science in 2001 I interviewed Professor Sashi Sashidharan, a senior psychiatrist who helped the UK Government to assess the state of mental health services for black and minority people. In his view, many white, British psychiatrists had long assumed that south Asian people living in the UK had low rates of depression compared to the general population. However, he had reviewed the recent research evidence, which was to the contrary.[19] He argued that the assumption that rates of prevalence of depression in these communities were relatively low was based on a cultural stereotype – a belief that south Asian people enjoy greater availability of support from extended family networks. However, much of what a white, middle-class, western psychiatrist knows about ethnic minority groups is derived from racial mythology, stereotyped images from the media, and images of these groups' countries of origin.[20]

In reality, traditional south Asian support networks can be a hindrance rather than a help, particularly if you are female and caught between cultures. In any case, many of the traditional support systems are breaking down. During a visit to a specialist Asian mental health service in Coventry, I met an elderly woman with depression. She told me that the obligation on the young to help the old is increasingly not being fulfilled in the UK as the young become more independent. The staff told me that this was indeed a trend that seemed to be increasing the rate of depression in the elderly Indian population.[21]

Observer bias is not only influenced by an expectation of low prevalence, however. Studies have been carried out that demonstrate that the person who asks questions about symptoms plays a significant role in what is reported. This is common sense. If a physician or psychiatrist in a non-western culture does not systematically ask about psychic symptoms of depression they will be missed, and the rate of depression will appear artificially low. The erroneous conclusion will be made that Africans and the Chinese, for example, present with only somatic symptoms when they are depressed (disproved by Beiser, among others).[13]

A research study carried out in Italy and Sweden in 1981 demonstrated how medical interviews are biased to reflect the prevailing attitudes of the profession and the society at large.[22] At that time, depressed Italians were thought to present with more hypochondriacal symptoms (focusing on physical complaints), whereas Swedish depressed patients were thought typically to present with restlessness and an inability to feel. In the two centres of Naples and Umea, the researchers compared the results of ratings of mental symptoms in depressed psychiatric inpatients *completed by physicians* with those made *by the patients themselves*, on a self-report questionnaire. The doctors' ratings were in line with each society's expectations. However, Swedish *self*-ratings actually yielded higher ratings of disturbance in bodily function than the Italians' ratings. Also, the Italians expressed more feelings of hopelessness and lack of interest than the Swedes, contradicting the idea that the Swedes were more in touch with their feelings and were less likely to somatise.

The culturally defined relationship between doctor and patient, and locally defined ideas of what is considered to be acceptable illness behaviour, will determine whether depression is detected and treated or not. Thus, it is far more acceptable for a patient to consult a doctor with feelings of despair and low self-esteem in the US than it would be in China or Japan, where the expression of emotion in front of an authority figure is taboo. Kleinman revealed a high proportion of depression in patients attending a Chinese clinic for the treatment of nervous exhaustion.[23] Physical symptoms had been used to negotiate care – and this was not necessarily different from the treatment for what westerners would call depression.

Complaints about *feeling* depressed do not regularly enter into physician–patient consultations in Africa, either. Again, different ideas prevail about what is legitimate to bring into a treatment encounter. In China and Africa mental distress can occasionally be discussed with family or close friends, healers, or fortune tellers, but is not considered appropriate subject matter for the medical consultation. By contrast, the majority culture in North America regards the disclosure of psychic distress within the patient–physician encounter as more acceptable.

Thus, results from community surveys vary widely. A survey in Bengal, eastern India, estimated the point prevalence to be 4.7 per cent, a figure not too different from estimates of prevalence in the west.[24] However, rates in North and South India have been reported to be 8.9 per cent and 3.3 per cent respectively.[25] Some field studies in West Bengal have recorded a prevalence of depression as high as 77.2 per cent in one village.[26] This figure seems improbably high.

WHO figures suggest that nearly four million elderly persons are mentally ill, and two-thirds of this morbidity is accounted for by mood disorders, predominantly depression.[27] According to one estimate, the prevalence of depression in the elderly of India at any one time is between 13 per cent and 22 per cent.[28] The main risk factors for depression in India are similar to those in the west; loss of fortune, fall in self-esteem, sense of helplessness, poor education, substandard physical health, social and sex discrimination, financial debt and status as a widowed person. Most of the depression goes undetected and/or untreated, as with the south Asian immigrant communities in the UK. Depression, therefore, is said to make a significant contribution to the overall burden of disability in the Indian subcontinent.[29]

Similar findings are emerging in other continents. Following improvements in survey techniques, Africans are now thought to have a prevalence of depression that is comparable to the rate observed in the UK.[30]

Depression was once considered uncommon in Arab countries. However an incidence of 24.5 per cent was reported in hospital outpatients in Egypt.[31] Depression most commonly presented in middle-aged housewives. A researcher called Pfeiffer, who originally reported a low figure for depression in Indonesia in the 1960s, later revised his position, and concluded that the WHO definition of depression occurs in significant numbers of Indonesians. [32,33]

In his review, Wolpert concludes that the rates for depression in the Far East are consistently less than 50 per cent of those in the west.[34] It is not clear why this should be so, but the perceived need of depressed people to negotiate care on the grounds of physical illness may be responsible for cases being missed.

The question of whether similar drug treatments are effective in alleviating depression in both the developed and developing worlds has been explored by Dr Venkoba Rao, an expert on transcultural psychiatry who is based in India.[35] It seems that similar drug treatments are equally effective in the UK and in India. There are similar rates of chronic, unresolved depression (i.e. treatment failures) and recurring depression. This supports the idea of a common biological mechanism for the condition around the globe.

The International Consortium of Psychiatric Epidemiology (ICPE) was established in 1998 by the WHO in an attempt to overcome limitations in cross-national survey techniques. The Composite International Diagnostic Interview (CIDI) was thought to be a valid and reliable measure – meaning that it detected what it was supposed to detect (depression) and that it would give the same result when used a number of times with the same depressed person by different interviewers.[36] It was like the SADD but it was designed to be used with patients in the community. At the turn of the new millennium a WHO Bulletin published the results of international comparisons using the CIDI.

In total 30,000 people were surveyed. All interviews were carried out face to face, not by telephone or by post. The results for mood

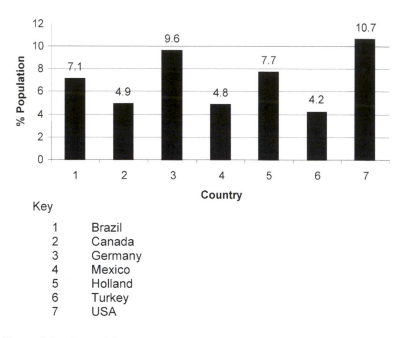

Key

1	Brazil
2	Canada
3	Germany
4	Mexico
5	Holland
6	Turkey
7	USA

Figure 3.2 Cases of depression over previous 12 months

disorders are shown in Figure 3.2. Mood disorders included depression, dysthymia (depressive personality) and/or mania, but major depression accounted for the greatest proportion of cases.

It is difficult to make meaningful comparisons from these figures alone because depression was not the only condition studied and the samples of the populations may not have accurately represented all people in every country. What we can conclude, however, is that the figures reveal a significant amount of depression in each country studied.

Overall, the weight of evidence from modern prevalence studies seems to show that the happy savage idea is untenable. The idea that traditional communities are immune from depression because, for example, they have less responsibility, they give greater expression to sadness and grieving, they have not developed the capacity for sadness, they are less psychologically minded, or they do not experience the same kind of stress, cannot be substantiated by the evidence collected so far. Depression, when carefully defined and carefully observed, appears to be a universal phenomenon.

The universality of grief – and its relationship to depression

Mourning rituals are observed in all the cultures of the globe. Most mourning rituals facilitate an effective channelling of grief into a socially acceptable pattern of behaviour that does not disrupt the group as a whole. Full cathartic expression is allowed within a carefully designed ritual, and within a defined context. Grief, therefore, is a common and universal human characteristic.[37]

It is worth pointing out that, from a psychiatrist's point of view, there appears to be a marked overlap between the syndromes of depression and grief. This overlap exists not only in terms of triggers, but also in terms of subjective experience, and duration of illness.

Depression is, after all, often diagnosed following bereavement. Conversely, grief reactions are increasingly diagnosed following other losses. With regard to symptoms, both grief and depression can present with poor sleep, poor appetite, lack of motivation, a lack of energy and reduced pleasure in sex and other activities. The symptoms endured during acute grief can be just as severe as those experienced during a depression. There seems to be just as much variation in the way grief presents itself as in the way depression presents itself. It can be argued that if depression were fundamentally a different phenomenon from grief, then our experiences of both would not be so similar. With regard to duration, depression is traditionally thought to last longer than grief. However, people with persistent depressive symptoms following bereavement often acquire a diagnosis of 'pathological grief', rather than depressive illness. Furthermore, depression does not need to be prolonged to be diagnosed.

Such diagnostic confusion might invite us to consider the possibility that we prefer to adopt the grief label in cases of depression following a loss because of social stigma. The term 'grief' is, after all, much more socially acceptable than the term 'depression'. If we had a generic term for all grief and all depression, if we considered both conditions together, we might then be more willing to accept that depression is a ubiquitous feature of human experience. Separation of the two conditions seems to be arbitrary. There is, at the very least, an overlap.

The universal nature of depression suggests that it is not an entirely culturally derived phenomenon. Culture will inevitably have some influence on the number of new cases of depression in a society, and on how long people remain depressed (which affects its prevalence at any one time), but it seems unlikely that the high rate of depression seen across different cultures around the world can be explained entirely in terms of a mismatch between culture and inherited brain biology. If this were the case, the prevalence of depression in more traditional cultures, where the mismatch is minimal, would be closer to zero. The idea that our propensity to depression is an evolved biological tendency in its own right is starting to look more viable. If we could demonstrate some continuity with other animals with regard to depressive behaviour then this would strengthen such a position even further. Darwin suggested that we share the tears of sorrow with other mammals.[1] Could it be that we have also inherited the capacity for depression from animals further down the evolutionary tree?

References

1 Darwin C. *The expression of the emotions in animals and man.* 3rd ed. London: Harper Collins; 1999.

2 Darwin C. *The origin of species.* New York: Gramercy Books; 1998.

3 Mead M. *Sex and temperament in three societies.* London: Harper Collins; 2001.

4 Goodenough FL. Expressions of the emotions in a blind–deaf child. *Journal of Abnormal and Social Psychology.* 1932; **27**: 328–33.

5 Thompson J. Development of facial expression of emotion in blind and seeing children. *Archives of Psychology.* 1941; **37**: No. 264.

6 Eibl-Eibesfeldt I. The expressive behaviour of the deaf-and-blind-born. In: von Cranach M, Vine I editors. *Social communication and movement.* London: Academic Press; 1973, p. 163–194.

7 Fulcher JS. 'Voluntary' facial expressions in blind and seeing children. *Archives of Psychology.* 1942; **38**: No. 272.

8 Freedman DG. Smiling in blind infants and the issue of innate versus acquired. *Journal of Child Psychology and Psychiatry.* 1964; **5**: 171–184.

9 Ekman P. *Darwin and facial expression.* Burlington, USA: Academic Press; 1973.

10 Sartorius N et al. *Depressive disorders in different cultures: report on the World Health Organization collaborative study on standardized assessment of depressive disorders.* Geneva: World Health Organization; 1983.

11 Majodina MZ and Johnson AFW. Standardized assessment of depressive disorder in Ghana. *British Journal of Psychiatry.* 1983; **143**: 442–6.

12 Kleinman A and Good B. *Culture and depression : studies in the anthropology and cross-cultural psychiatry of affect and disorder.* Berkeley: University of California Press; 1985.

13 Beiser M, Burr WA, Ravel JL *et al.* Illnesses of the spirit among the Serer of Senegal. *American Journal of Psychiatry.* 1973; **130**: 881–5.

14 Wittkower ED. Perspectives in transcultural psychiatry. *International Journal of Psychiatry.* 1969; **8**: 811–24.

15 Carrothers JC. A study of mental derangement in Africans and an attempt to explain its peculiarities more especially in relation to the African attitude to life. *Journal of Mental Science.* 1947; **83**: 548–97.

16 Kraepelin E. Psychiatrisches aus Java. *Cbl Nervenheilk Psychiatrie.* 1904; **27**: 468–9.

17 Shaw WS. *Clinical Handbook of Mental Diseases.* Calcutta: Butterworth and Co.; 1925.

18 Kakar SJ. Psychoanalysis and Eastern spiritual healing traditions. *Analytische Psychologie.* 2003; **48**: 659–78.

19 Commander MJ, Cochrane R, Sashidharan SP *et al.* Mental health care for Asian, black and white patients with non-affective psychoses: pathways to the psychiatric hospital, in-patient and after-care. *Social Psychiatry and Psychiatric Epidemiology.* 1999; **34**: 484–91.

20 Sashidharan SP and Francis E. Racism in psychiatry necessitates reappraisal of general procedures and Eurocentric theories. *British Medical Journal.* 1999; **319**: 254.

21 Reid-Galloway C. *The mental health of the South Asian community in Britain.* Mind Information Unit, Mind Publications; 2000. www.mind.org.uk (accessed 17 July 2006).

22 Perris C, Eisemann M, Eriksson U *et al.* Transcultural aspects of depressive symptomatology. *Psychiatrica Clinica.* 1981; **14**: 69–80.

23 Kleinman A. *Social origins of distress and disease: depression, neurasthenia, and pain in modern China.* New Haven: Yale University Press; 1986.

24 Carstairs GM and Kapur RL. *The great universe of Kota: stress changes and mental disorders in an Indian village.* London: Hogarth Press; 1976.

25 Sethi BB, Nathawat SS and Gupta SC. Depression in India. *Journal of Social Psychology.* 1973; **91**: 3.

26 Nandi DN, Banerjee G, Nandi S *et al.* Is hysteria on the wane? A community survey in West Bengal, India. *British Journal of Psychiatry.* 1992; **160**: 87–91.

27 WHO Consortium in Psychiatric Epidemiology. Cross-national comparisons of the prevalences and correlates of mental disorders. *Bulletin of the World Health Organization.* 2000; **78**: 413–26.

28 Joshi PC and Sengupta SN. Health Issues. In: *Seminar 488: Ageing; a symposium on the greying of our society.* Seminar (on line). 2000.

29 Rao AV. Mental health and ageing in India. *Indian Journal of Psychiatry.* 1981; **23**: 11–20.

30 German GA. Mental health in Africa: I. The extent of mental health problems in Africa today. An update of epidemiological knowledge. *British Journal of Psychiatry.* 1987; **151**: 435–9.

31 Okasha A. Psychiatric symptomatology in Egypt. *Mental Health and Society.* 1977; **4**: 121–5.

32 Pfeiffer WM. States of torpor and trance in Indonesian tribes. *Nervenarzt.* 1966; **37**: 7–18.

33 Pfeiffer WM. Cross-cultural psychiatry. *Deutsch Krankenpflegez.* 1975; **28**: 547–50.

34 Wolpert L. *Malignant sadness. The anatomy of depression.* London: Faber and Faber; 2001.

35 Rao AV. Psychiatry for the developing world. In: Tantum D, Duncan A. Appleby L, editors. London: Gaskell, p. 187–221.

36 Andrews G and Peters L. The psychometric properties of the Composite International Diagnostic Interview. *Social Psychiatry and Psychiatric Epidemiology.* 1998; **33**: 80–8.

37 Triandis HC and Draguns JG, editors. *Handbook of cross-cultural psychology. Vol. 6.* London: Allyn and Bacon; 2005.

CHAPTER 4

Depression's place in the animal kingdom

Darwin's theory of evolution is the best theory we have to explain the nature of our animal kingdom.[1] This one unifying theory explains how apparently beneficial change takes place in life forms over many generations, how seemingly close anatomical relationships exist between different animals (the hand, the flipper and the wing, for example) and how the seemingly purposeful quality of the giraffe's long neck or the woodpecker's beak could have come about. If we accept Darwin's theory then we must accept that we have descended from other mammals. If animals get depressed then it follows that we may have inherited a biological basis for depression that is older than humanity. Darwin once said 'the major part [of our emotions], *presumably including depression* [my italics], are due to historical antecedents registered in the susceptible organisms. No experience of the individual can account for the strength or direction of feeling'. In other words, there is something built into the brain, an emotional programme, which has been inherited from other susceptible mammals.

The map of the human brain was not drawn on a blank canvas. The evolution of the hominid has resulted in extra layers being added to the brains of animals further down the evolutionary tree. Let us consider Paul MacLean's model of the 'triune brain' (see Figure 4.1), which proposes that the human brain consists of three fairly well-delineated archetypal sub-brains, each fitting round the other like parts of a Russian doll.[2,3] These brains consist of the 'reptilian' brain, the 'paleo-mammalian' brain and the 'neo-mammalian' brain.

The reptilian part of our brains developed 300 million years ago, when we crawled out of the oceans, and we share this structure with most vertebrates. The reptilian brain controls the functions essential for vertebrate life, like breathing air. It also controls certain basic types

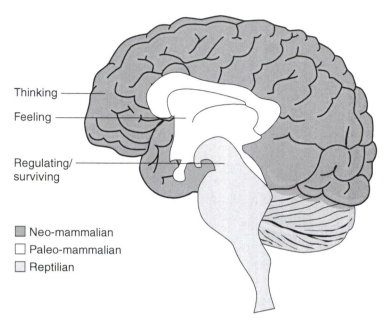

Thinking

Feeling

Regulating/
surviving

■ Neo-mammalian
□ Paleo-mammalian
□ Reptilian

Figure 4.1 The triune brain (after Maclean)

of behaviour – like defending territory and mating – that are largely instinctive, automatic, or even compulsive. Freud might have suggested that the 'id' – a slave to our drives to defend ourselves and reproduce – was contained within this brain layer.[4,5] The seductively labelled 'R-Complex' can override our moral codes of conduct, causing us to act impulsively, perhaps even deceptively, in order to fulfil a basic need; thus, we sometimes behave in ways that our higher cortical centres cause us to despise.[6]

The next layer – our paleo-mammalian layer – is seen in animals higher up the evolutionary tree: it is a feature of all mammals. The paleo-mammalian brain has evolved a feelings centre known as the limbic system, connected to a body control centre called the hypothalamus. This system not only helps to keep our body's internal state fairly constant – balancing hunger with satiation, thirst with fluid retention, and causing us to sweat when we're hot, shiver when we're cold and so on – it also controls our emotions. At this stage of brain evolution it is now possible to experience fear, anger, love, attachment and bonding. Behaviours like nursing and maternal care, the separation call of the infant, and the capacity to engage in play all help to distinguish the mammal from the reptile – and the limbic system makes such behaviour possible. Behaviour at this level is less of a slave to instinct. However, at this stage of evolution, there is still a lack of capacity to attach meaning to events.

The cold, calculating, cognitive brain is located in the next layer – the neo-mammalian brain. This rational brain acts as moderator, reining in the instinctive and emotional impulses, so that we may cooperate more effectively with other members of our social group. Freud might have placed the 'super-ego' in this layer.[4,5] In the neo-mammalian brain events can be compared with our internal working models of the world so that we can attach meaning to them. Deduction and problem solving are possible. Memory traces of past experience contribute to our working models of the world and help us to predict the outcome of events. Functions of the neo-mammalian brain are seen in high-order mammals, like apes, and humans. When we are drunk this part of the brain is subdued, and we become servants of our more primitive brain layers.

Humans, who are quintessentially social animals, have further developed the neocortex, particularly the frontal lobes. We are masters at predicting behaviour in complex social situations, and we have developed an extensive theory of mind function – an ability to anticipate how others might be thinking or feeling. This ability is diminished or absent in people on the autistic spectrum, and hence autistic people never develop normal empathy. Psychopathic people are also said to lack empathy, although, unlike autistic people, they can manipulate others with superficial charm and Machiavellian tears, but they are usually found out, and become imprisoned or ostracised. True compassion and empathy are essential for normal human functioning because we are interdependent – we have to rely on our neighbour to help us raise children, to care for us when we are young, sick or infirm, to help protect us from enemies, to pay us money, or, in the past, to share the results of the hunt. The higher cortical centres help us to develop these important social skills throughout life. A special anatomical feature of the human brain that is not seen in lower-order mammals is an extensive lateralisation of function. If you are right-handed you may use the left side of your brain mostly for deduction and language production, reserving the right side for more creative thinking, control of mood, and so on.

So, the human brain has developed by adding new functions to previous functions. This is how evolution works. It is possible that depression emerged in higher order mammals as a result of an inter-action between the thinking brain and the feeling brain – the neocortex and the limbic system. It may be the result of a circular feedback between the higher centres and the lower ones. Is there any evidence to suggest that depression is a feature of not just the human brain but of the mammalian brain in general?

The depressed primate

Primates and humans share 98 per cent of their DNA. They also share a lot of behaviours, like playing, mother–infant bonding, and nurturing. Pertinent to the current issue is how similarly they react to interpersonal separation, particularly infant–mother separation, and to any prolonged threat or stress.

After being deserted by their mothers, infant chimpanzees and monkeys whimper and cry with distress just like human infants. Also, as seen in human infants, this 'protest phase' will progress, if the separation is prolonged for several days, to a 'despair phase'. During the despair phase the infant rhesus or pig-tailed macaque sits hunched and alone with its head held low. It no longer plays with the rest of the group. The despairing monkey looks very similar to the despairing human infant. To the human observer, the most convincing similarity is the characteristic drooping mouth, perhaps the closest link that we have to our hairy ancestors when looking for correlates of depression (see Figure 4.2). Darwin first noted these similarities over 130 years ago.[7]

The striking similarities between the two sequential responses to early separation in humans, apes and monkeys – a period of agitated yearning followed by a period of withdrawal and relative inactivity – suggest that the mediating biological mechanisms are common to all these species (see Box 4.1). Consequently, it is believed that the two reactions are probably innate, and share a common genetic lineage.[8]

It has also been shown that the risk of developing the depressive despair reaction to separation can be reduced in young animals if adequate surrogate care is provided by another nurturing adult.[8] In one experiment, infant pig-tailed macaques, who had been separated from their immediate caregivers but received some comfort from other adults, did not go through a despair phase. Conversely, in another experiment, a bonnet macaque did become depressed when left alone in its cage with pig-tailed monkeys which showed absolutely no concern for it.

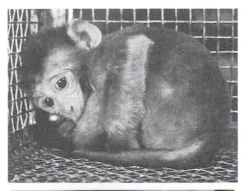

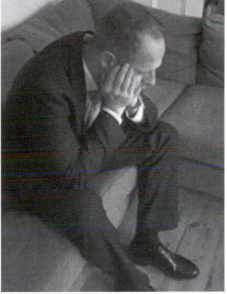

Figure 4.2 The depressed monkey (From Chamove AS. The effects of varying infant peer experience on social behaviour in the rhesus monkey. Unpublished MA Thesis, University of Wisconsin, 1996.) and the depressed man

Similarly, in humans, abandoned children who are placed with good foster carers have some protection against the despair response, particularly if the foster carer was known to the child before separation from the biological parents. Any strong substitute attachment can be protective against a depressive reaction in the short and long term. Separation from a parent or the loss of a parent in early childhood,

Box 4.1   Biology and separation
There is additional evidence in support of a common underlying biological mechanism at play. It has been observed, for example, that both humans and primates have raised levels of a chemical called cortisol in their blood during the protest phase of separation.[9] Although the functions of this chemical are not completely understood, we know that it is released into the blood in response to stress, and that this helps to prepare the body to meet a challenge to its survival. The size of this cortisol response predicts a greater intensity of the depressive response during the subsequent despair phase. There are also well-recognised abnormalities of brain chemistry in the despair phase that are not present during the protest phase. There is a reduction in the brain chemical serotonin, for example, which can be prevented with antidepressant medication.[10]

without the provision of adequate substitute care, seems to leave a psychological imprint, an implicit emotional memory, which can be reactivated by other interpersonal separations when the unfortunate child grows up. Separations or bereavements in adulthood are more likely to lead to depression, or abnormally prolonged grief, in those who have experienced a loss or separation (without any alternative attachment of quality) during their formative years. Adequate maternal care, or a good substitute, seems to be essential for the normal emotional development of the social mammal in its early years, and this facilitates the forming of strong attachments to others in the future. In other words, a good early relationship will lead to successful adult relationships.

We know that, in the human adult, depression can be triggered by the loss of someone close (after bereavement or divorce), but this will look different from the infant reaction to the loss of a parent because it is modified by brain maturation, learning and experience. What is the evidence that older animals react in a similar way to these types of separation?

A lot of evidence comes from observing animals in zoos.[11] In 1930, a zoologist called Zedtwitz famously observed the behaviour of an adult female orang-utan called Cleo, whose first mate had died of tuberculosis. For most of the day, day in day out, Cleo would remain in her sleeping box, inanimate, wrapped in a rug. Occasionally she would venture toward the heating lamp and sit under it with bowed head and downcast mouth. In 1954, an eight-month-old baby gorilla was observed for abnormal behaviours after it had been separated from its family in the wild and placed in Antwerp Zoo. It was noted that it was indifferent when a young chimpanzee was introduced to its cage. It would not eat when offered food in a bottle, and lost weight. Only 20 days later did it begin taking adequate amounts of nourishment, and start to improve.

It has been suggested that some zoo animals can show no overt signs of depression but, at post-mortem, have internal lesions indicative of chronic stress and adrenal exhaustion due to the excessive release of stress hormone. Just as man may attempt to mask his depression to maintain acceptance in his social milieu, certain animals, notably wallabies and kangaroos, maintain normal overt behaviour to ensure acceptance by other members of the herd, and to escape the notice of predators.[12]

Dr Brunner was one of the first veterinary researchers to observe and record the effects of separation on cats and dogs who were kennelled when the owners went on holiday: 'The pet refuses to eat and withdraws into a dark corner of the kennel or cage . . . the animal is hypoactive [less active], but may remain tense and constantly alert.'[13] He believed that the pets were experiencing 'acute depression', and suggested that this reaction could provide 'a useful model for the study of depression in man'. It was possible to prevent this depression in kennels or catteries by bringing some object from the pet's home such as a toy, the animal's basket, or some piece of clothing. Comparisons can be made with the reactions of infant humans who are separated from their parents when they are admitted to hospital. They are similarly reassured by items such as the comfort blanket that are taken from home to hospital.

Many other similar cases have been published. Horses typically '[go] down and give up' after a relatively trivial infection or injury if they have been moved from one paddock to another. While assisting in an animal psychology consulting centre in Vienna, Dr F Brunner witnessed the behaviour of a Dobermann pinscher and a German boxer, after they had lost close companions. The Dobermann had started to act abnormally 24 hours after the death of a tomcat 'with which the dog grew up and shared sleeping quarters'. From an early age the dog had defended the cat from the more hostile attention of less familiar dogs. Just one day after the death of the cat the dog had started to refuse food. It was 'no longer playful; it would wait at the front door, search the room, and was generally listless'. These behavioural changes went on for the next two weeks. When the Dobermann was tranquillised and moved with the same owner to a different location, its behaviour returned to normal over the course of three weeks.

The German boxer began to behave in a depressed fashion after the death of its master, who had lived with the dog continuously for nine years, since the dog had been only two months old. The boxer 'paced during the night, lacked an appetite, and lost weight, was listless, apathetic, and showed no guarding behaviour when strangers knocked on the door'. By the time the unfortunate animal had been brought to the attention of Dr Brunner and his colleagues, it had been behaving in this way for three whole months. Sadly, tranquillisation had no effect on this dog, and it died two months later from uncertain causes.

Chronic stress and learned helplessness

Not all human adult depression arises from separation. It can arise in the context of any chronic life difficulty that has a long-term impact on wellbeing.

Social scientists have shown that depression is more likely to follow a negative life event if the event leads to a persisting sense of impending disaster or humiliation – otherwise known as an environment of 'chronic threat'.[14] A chronic threat could be a financial burden, with a persistent threat of eviction, a battle over access to children following a divorce, a feeling of being continually out of one's depth at work, trying to raise children without help, clinging on to a dying relationship, or the threat of violent assault from a spouse. By implication, there is a sense of 'entrapment' – a feeling that one is powerless to escape the stressful life conditions. Negative events, like bereavement, can, of course, occur on top of an existing chronic life difficulty – like marital conflict – and this will make us more vulnerable also.

If a problem is causing anxiety the mind is designed to work overtime to find a solution, but sometimes no clear solution is forthcoming. The failure to find a solution causes more anxiety, which then prompts more cognitive effort, and so on, in a vicious cycle. It seems that these escalating ruminations can tip us into depression if they persist for too long. People who have a particularly ruminatory coping style, including Marco, may be more susceptible. Such people tend to be more self-analytical, reflective, introverted. Extroverts, conversely, are less prone.

It seems that an organism can only tolerate so much potential threat before it gives up expending energy – as if it reaches some point of stress-induced exhaustion. If you subject any mammal to inescapable electric shocks, or force it to swim in a confined area, it will eventually adopt a state of inanimation: in each respective situation it will either stay still and be shocked, or it will stop swimming and float. Adopting a state of inanimation seems like a sensible strategy, but when the animal is subsequently given the opportunity to escape it will maintain its inanimate state.

This phenomenon of persistent inactivity and lack of motivation was first described by the psychologist Martin Seligman, of the University of Pennsylvania, who coined the term 'learned helplessness'.[15] He suggested that if, over a protracted period of time, all attempts to escape from a stressful situation prove to be futile we will stop trying to escape because we have learnt that we are helpless to change our circumstance. However, it seems more likely that this is a biological reaction which occurs automatically, without a conscious learning process. How quickly it comes about, and how long it lasts, will depend on the biological make-up of the organism, possibly influenced by genes.

Seligman was quick to draw comparisons between this persistent inanimate state in animals and the type of human depression that is brought about by inescapable life difficulties.[16] Animals with learned helplessness demonstrate behavioural changes that are similar to those seen in human depression. Helpless animals show reduced bodily activity, less motivation to eat, loss of weight, reduced sleep and early wakening. Although there is considerable variability (possibly under genetic control) in how long the helplessness lasts in animals, the effects have been found in some studies to last for up to several months, which is comparable to the length of a depressive episode in humans.[17,18] Further evidence has emerged of similarities between helplessness in animals and human depression. There are changes in the brain chemistry – such as a reduction in serotonin and noradrenaline turnover, which are also seen in human depression.[19,20] Moreover, the moribund state can be prematurely reversed with antidepressants, as with human depression. Also, the onset of learned helplessness in rats who have been forced to swim in a confined space has been delayed by treating them in advance with these drugs.[17,18]

Thus, we can argue that Seligman's experiments provide a model of depression that applies to both humans and animals. Rather than being learned, the depressive response may be an old and instinctive biological mechanism, which is activated following any protracted, but ultimately futile, stress response, otherwise known as the 'fight or flight' response.[21] We automatically engage this potentially helpful response in the face of a life challenge – like entering a race, attending a job interview, having an argument with a loved one, or confronting an enemy. This adrenaline-charged state prepares our bodies for action so that we can meet the challenge effectively. Blood flow is directed to the brain and the skeletal muscles. We become more alert, more sensitive to noise.

States of heightened arousal will be accompanied by emotions of fear, anger, jealousy, sadness and so on, depending on the context. These emotional reactions have the potential to trigger depression if they are excessive and prolonged.

The lack of a fully developed symbolic language in animals will, of course, always limit our interpretation of their mood states. We have to rely on behaviour rather than subjective account, and our own emotional reactions to their behaviour influence our interpretations.

Nevertheless, a similar depressive-style reaction (at least in terms of observable changes in behaviour and biology) appears to occur in both animals and humans in response to similar stresses. These include separation, removal to an unfamiliar environment, and entrapment in a stressful environment. Furthermore, humans and other mammals appear to share the same protective factors following separations – like a familiar object, or a surrogate carer.

The depressive-type reaction appears to be similar in all mammals, which implies a common brain mechanism and a common genetic blueprint. Therefore it is probable that depression is as old as humanity itself, having been inherited from the other social mammals who are our distant ancestors.

References

1 Darwin C. *The origin of species.* New York: Gramercy Books; 1998.

2 MacLean PD. *A triune concept of the brain and behaviour.* Toronto: University of Toronto Press; 1973.

3 MacLean PD. Evolutionary psychiatry and the triune brain. *Psychological Medicine.* 1985; **15**: 219–21.

4 Freud S. *The ego and the id.* New York: Norton; 1923.

5 Young A. Remembering the evolutionary Freud. *Science in Context.* 2006; **19**: 175–89.

6 Bailey K. *Human paleopsychology: applications to aggression and pathological processes.* Hillsdale, NJ: Lawrence Erlbaum Associates; 1987.

7 Darwin C. *The expression of the emotions in animals and man.* 3rd ed. London: Harper Collins; 1999.

8 Passingham RE. *The human primate.* Oxford and San Francisco: Freeman and Co; 1982.

9 Higley JD, Suomi SJ, Scanlon JM *et al.* Plasma cortisol as a predictor of individual depressive behaviour in rhesus monkeys (Macaca mulatta). *Abstracts – Society for Neuroscience.* 1982; **8**: 461.

10 Levine S, Johnson DF, Gonzalez CA. Behavioral and hormonal responses to separation in infant rhesus monkeys and mothers. *Behavioral Neuroscience.* 1985; **99**: 399–410.

11 Meyer-Holzapfel M. Abnormal behaviour in zoo animals. In: Fox MW, editor. *Abnormal behaviour in animals.* Philadelphia: Saunders; 1968, p. 476–503.

12 Fox MW. Psychomotor disturbances. In: Fox MW, editor. *Abnormal behaviour in animals.* Philadelphia: Saunders; 1968, p. 357–45.

13 Brunner F. The application of behaviour studies in small animal practice. In: Fox MW, editor. *Abnormal behaviour in animals.* Philadelphia: Saunders; 1968, p.398–449.

14 Kendler KS, Hettema JM, Butera F *et al.* Life event dimensions of loss, humiliation, entrapment, and danger in the prediction of onsets of major depression and generalized anxiety. *Archives of General Psychiatry.* 2003; **60**: 789–96.

15 Seligman ME. Learned helplessness. *Annual Review of Medicine.* 1972; **23**: 407–12.

16 Miller WR, Seligman ME. Depression and learned helplessness in man. *Journal of Abnormal Psychology.* 1975; **84**: 228–38.

17 Willner P. The validity of animal models of depression. *Psychopharmacology.* 1984; **83**: 1–16.

18 Willner P. Validation criteria for animal models of human mental disorders: learned helplessness as a paradigm case. *Progress in Neuropsychopharmacology and Biological Psychiatry.* 1986; **10**: 677–690.

19 Weiss JM, Simson PE. Neurochemical and electrophysiological events underlying stress-induced depression in an animal model. *Advances in Exerimental Medicine and Biology.* 1988; **245**: 425–440.

20 Kirby LG, Chou-Green JM, Davis K *et al.* The effects of different stressors on extracellular 5-hydroxytryptamine and 5-hydroxyindoleacetic acid. *Brain Research.* 1997; **760**:218–230.

21 Cannon WB. *Bodily changes in pain, hunger, fear and rage.* 2nd ed. New York: Appleton; 1929.

CHAPTER 5

Adaptation or fluff?

Why did depression persist in our ancestors' environment? Given the apparent lack of competitiveness associated with being in the state of depression, why didn't human brains adapt? In other words, why haven't the depression genes been bred out? Why has our brain biology allowed depression to persist? Let's examine all the possible explanations.

The imperfect adaptation

First, depression may be an adaptation, which is the main idea that we are trying to test.

If depression were an adaptation it would not be a perfect adaptation. No adaptation is. Adaptations are always a compromise between benefits and costs.[1] Whether the benefits of experiencing a depressive illness have outweighed the costs, in terms of fitness, is the bottom line in determining whether or not depression is an adaptation.

Adaptations are imperfect because they are not created from scratch: they have to improve on what went before.

If we consider the human spine we recall that it has evolved from a structure designed for walking on all fours. It is a compromise. Most doctors will tell us that the spine of *Homo erectus* is poorly designed for walking upright. Back pain is the single most common cause of time off work and it is responsible for a huge number of visits to the family doctor. Orthopaedic surgeons could probably suggest much more robust designs if they were able to start with a blank drawing board. There are costs attached to walking erect – arthritis, slipped discs and so on – that are in balance with the benefits. On average, however, the benefits of walking upright have probably outweighed the costs over the course of our evolutionary history.[2] An erect spine would have given man a better view for hunting and for spotting approaching predators. It would have made it easier for him to make and use tools. Of course, evolution has not ended in the twenty-first century. The human spine may acquire further refinements in the future, which may lead to fewer problems.

Sometimes evolved mechanisms have really marked costs. If, on first viewing, we saw a giraffe struggling to drink from a water hole, we might conclude that the poor creature had been afflicted by a terrible handicap, some awful mutation which made it difficult for it to bend over. If, however, we were to dispense with our initial prejudice and start looking for advantages, we would notice that that same giraffe can also eat leaves from a tall tree. This is pretty useful in the savannah, where food is literally thin on the ground. Suddenly we realise: the advantages of the long neck outweigh the disadvantages.

Some people, like Randolphe Nesse, professor of academic affairs in the department of psychiatry, University of Michigan School of Medicine, who coined the phrase 'Darwinian medicine', have proposed that this compensation is a feature of people's phobias.[3] There are clear survival advantages to fearing snakes, spiders, confined and crowded places, or heights. In some people the fear becomes excessive and irrational, and is apparently handicapping. However, Nesse would say that it is better to have 100 false alarms than to receive one fatal injury – the so-called 'smoke detector principle'.[4] Studies conducted in accident and emergency departments of large hospitals have suggested that people with anxiety disorders might actually have fewer accidents than everyone else.

It has also been proposed that male sexual jealousy is an adaptation.[5] Clearly there are potential costs as well as possible benefits. Although jealousy is associated with anger and may lead to confrontation, and therefore injury, it may also increase differential reproductive success by enforcing monogamy, at least up to a point. Monogamy may lead to more reliable opportunities to reproduce.

Depression as genetic fluff

A second possible reason for the persistence of depression relates to age. If depression occurred only in older people it would not affect reproductive success. Hence, it would not be amenable to gene selection and would persist irrespective of whether it was adaptive or not. However, this explanation can be discounted because depression seems to occur in people of all ages. (It is increasingly recognised that the rate of depression in young people is high).

A third possible reason for depression's persistence, that would be independent of any adaptive value, is the protection afforded by the rest of the social group or kinship. Social support and interdependence were important features of the ancestral environment.[6] The group could have offered extra help to the depressed person until the condition resolved. However, this alone seems to an insufficient explanation for depression persisting, because it seems logical that the lack of competitive ground lost during the depression would have had led to a selection bias unless there was some compensatory advantage. In any case, although early studies suggested that depression tends to elicit a caring response from others, recent evidence is more equivocal, suggesting that depressed people are criticised and shunned, especially if they remain depressed for a year or more.[7–10]

However, there may be a specific adaptive function that depression exerts on the social milieu, and that is bargaining for more help and support in the long term. A depressed person may change the attitudes of other people toward him, making them more sympathetic to his needs and therefore giving him a long term advantage. We will explore this possibility in the next chapter.

Finally, depression may have had no advantages in itself but may have persisted as a by-product of something so useful that it outweighed the costs of depression over the millennia. In other words depression could be just genetic 'fluff' (a term probably first coined by Buss).[1] This is an interesting idea, which needs to be explored. We need to try to rule out this notion before we can even start to explore the possible adaptive benefits of the condition, but first let's examine the by-product idea with a useful analogy.

A good example from the physical domain is the observation that resistance to malaria is associated with a blood disorder called 'sickle cell' anaemia, a genetic condition in which some red blood cells no longer form a round structure but distort into a sort of comma shape, rather like a sickle. This causes problems with getting oxygen to vulnerable organs in the body. It can cause organs sensitive to oxygen supply like the kidney to fail, it is painful, and it can be fatal. However, you can be a carrier of the disorder without being affected too badly. Those who are carriers tend to be more resistant to malaria. The reason for this is that, after someone has been bitten by an infected mosquito, malaria bugs (called protozoa) infect the red blood cells in order to move around the body. It is much more difficult for the malaria protozoa to invade a sickle cell than a healthy spherical blood cell. So, in malaria-endemic areas, there are much higher numbers of people with the genes for sickle cell anaemia than there are in non-endemic areas. This is the callous balance sheet of natural selection: you can either have an increased chance of dying from sickle cell anaemia or suffer an even greater risk of dying from malaria, which is still one of the world's biggest killers.

Language and thought

Returning to the human brain, as brain functions have become more complex the chances of them interacting in unpredictable and potentially harmful ways have increased. Some helpful brain functions may also activate unhelpful brain circuits.

Language development has been very important to the success of the human species. Depression might be an unhelpful by-product of this development, as has been argued for schizophrenia.[11] In other words, depression may have persisted, despite being of no inherent adaptive value, because the adaptive value of language has outweighed the costs of depression. With the growth of language we have developed a lateralisation of brain function, as highlighted in the last chapter. The brain has become more flexible and malleable. This has also allowed for more diverse and abstract patterns of thinking and greater intelligence alongside better communication. However, these characteristics, although advantageous, may make depression more likely.

Human language is very rich in symbols and abstract concepts compared with the language used by other animals. It is possible that we, as humans, are more susceptible to depression than animals because we are able to symbolise our emotional distress, describe it, and the causes for it, and then ruminate on those causes. Humans probably have a greater ability to ruminate about their own personal inadequacies than the rest of the animal kingdom. Also, humans may be uniquely placed to contemplate their own inevitable demise.

However, complex language could not have evolved before depression if we accept, as Darwin did, that humans acquired depression from their ancestral mammals.[12] It follows that if a link could be found between depression and the development of a complex language this would not explain the ultimate origin of depression; it would only explain how depression may be exacerbated, or how it may have become more common. Nevertheless, this is an interesting idea to explore.

Thought is influenced by the use of language. For example, memory for colours is determined by the availability of colour names.[13] Depressive thinking may similarly be influenced by the terms that we have developed to describe ourselves in relation to others. Such an idea would dovetail neatly with Beck's ideas on the importance of a negative thinking style (or 'negative cognitive set') in the generation of depression, and with the building evidence for a ruminatory coping style – brooding on one's misfortunes – as a predictor of depression.[14–16] The presumed origins of these problems lie in weak attachments, separations or abusive parenting in childhood which distort reality and lead to overly negative views of the self. Introspective people, liable to self-analysis, are more prone to depression, and this may be mediated by a tendency to ruminate.[17,18]

Although language may mediate the effects of adult vulnerability in this way, it is not likely to be necessary for the original development of that vulnerability in childhood. Clearly, the infant 'depressive' reaction to maternal separation is not language mediated, nor is the mechanism of learned helplessness in mammals, which seems to share so many features with human depression (see last chapter). Modern theories of vulnerability to depression provide biological evidence in mammals and humans for a disordered control of the stress response originating in the infant or child during parental abuse, stress or separation. This takes the form of abnormal levels of 'corticotrophin releasing hormone', which controls levels of the stress hormone cortisol. These abnormalities persist, which may make the adult more susceptible to subsequent stresses.[19] Neo-Freudians like Klein are unlikely to attach much importance to the use of language in the psychological origins of depression because the 'depressive position' is assumed to arise before the age of three.[20] Neuroscientists have suggested that toxic (stressful) environments experienced in infancy initially act by inducing plastic changes in the brain.[21] These changes are to be expressed as cognitive vulnerability later on, when language has developed sufficiently to facilitate negative self-analysis. In other words, the self-denigrating language associated with vulnerability to depression might occur largely *as a consequence* of biological changes occurring in early childhood. Such language is probably a result of the adult searching after a meaning for how he feels.

Children with depression do not express themselves in this way because they lack the same self-reflective sophistication. Hence, a child or adolescent can experience sadness and low self-esteem without being able to describe these experiences. In the case of recurrent depression occurring over a lifetime the illness often started in childhood, but is often only understood in retrospect by the grown adult who wonders why he did so badly in that school year. Admittedly depression before adolescence is relatively rare, but it exists in significant numbers of children. Childhood suicides are on the increase. Depression is often not detected in children because it is not looked for, and, of course, young children find it difficult to express how they feel. Child psychiatrists are now getting better at asking the right questions and, partly as a result of this, childhood depression appears to be on the increase.

Even in adulthood, language need not always interact with vulnerability to trigger depression. Some researchers have demonstrated an absence of negative thinking in formerly depressed individuals, arguing that Beck's cognitive distortions are a consequence of depression rather than a cause of it.[22] In reality both are probably true, and we will address this again in Chapter 7. An important piece of evidence which suggests that the manifestation of depression may be independent of the use of a sophisticated language is the fact that people with a low verbal IQ commonly become depressed.[23]

In any case, one could argue convincingly that language equally allows us to consider reasons to be positive about ourselves. If language has facilitated negative rumination, which has been shown to predispose to depression, it has also facilitated positive thinking and religious beliefs which may compensate for the negative effects. Some people are particularly good at putting a positive spin on misfortune, and they frequently avoid depression. Language helps them to do this.

Religious beliefs are ubiquitous in traditional tribes and they are still common in the modern western civilisations.[24] Dependent on a rich language, they can buffer against the onset of depression. Religion frequently provides solace for people in the face of suffering. On balance, religious people seem to experience less depression and unhappiness than non-believers.

Religion can bring added happiness to those people for whom life lacks meaning, by providing much-needed direction. People who lacked direction might have otherwise been prone to depression. In one study, 101 undergraduates, aged 18 to 45, completed measures of happiness, purpose in life and positive attitudes towards Christianity.[25] Although happiness was related to strong Christian beliefs, not all religious people were happy. Those religious people who were happier also had a strong sense of purpose to their lives.

Religion has probably evolved mainly due to a need to find extra resolve in dealing with seemingly insurmountable problems. Sometimes events seem out of our control, and seem to challenge us beyond our resources for coping. Nevertheless our brains have been designed to find solutions. It is difficult to sustain hope in these situations, and we suffer from unpleasant psychological symptoms, including despair, and, ultimately, depression. Praying to a higher spiritual being can give us added hope, particularly if we are feeling isolated or unloved. If we believe that a God loves us unconditionally, this can be a great source of strength in the face of adversity.

The act of praying may serve a unique function by engendering a sense of calm and connectedness during times of hardship. Prayer is reportedly a great comfort to a great many people. A study of prayer and psychological wellbeing among evangelical Christians, conducted in Southern California, attempted to gain an understanding of the impact that frequent praying might have on a client undergoing therapy.[26] The results revealed that those who prayed more frequently had higher ratings of happiness and purpose in life than those who prayed less frequently.

In summary, the genesis of depression in an individual appears to be largely independent of language. Furthermore, something very akin to depression, which manifests similar behaviour, biology, triggers and time course, is manifest in the mammals from whom we have evolved; they clearly lack the same facility for language. Therefore, depression is unlikely to represent the genetic fluff of language, or even highly developed intelligence.

Personality

The by-product idea could, instead, be replaced more usefully with the idea of 'compensatory' elements occurring in a predisposing personality trait. For example, we know that there is a link between 'neuroticism' and depression. Neuroticism has a heritability of about 50 per cent (meaning that genes are quite important). The genetic contribution to depression may be entirely mediated by personality type. This trait can be beneficial as well as problematic. For example, neuroticism is associated with competitive spirit and success. Consequently, if neuroticism persists because of these advantages, its link with depression means that depression might be more likely to persist also. The main problem with this theory, however, is that many depression sufferers did not have abnormal personalities prior to their illness, or at least not that we can reliably measure.

There are other technical challenges to the idea of depression as adaptation, including the 'failure' of natural selection in conditions coded for by many genes, and the 'developmental instability' model. Neither seem to stand up to scrutiny in the case of depression (see Box 5.1 and Box 5.2). In general then, it is worth considering the first possibility in a bit more detail – the idea that the common (mild to moderate) form of depression is, at least in part, an adaptation.

Box 5.1 The 'failure of natural selection'

It has been argued that any human characteristic that is coded for by many genes of small effect will not necessarily comply with the normal laws of natural selection for the very reason that the characteristic has a bell shaped curve of genetic vulnerability. So, for example, if our moods are controlled by many genes, some that are on the more 'depressive' end of the scale will always get through because they can be carried by unaffected individuals with enough 'resilience' genes to compensate. In other words, the 'tendency towards the mean' results in what we can term an 'adaptive middle ground' of moderate genetic vulnerability (the main part of the bell), with noise around the edges. This is a curious argument, but not a convincing one because depression is too common to be restricted to the population's edges. Any common characteristic coded for by a lot or a few genes will still comply with the phenomenon of genetic drift. In other words, genetic variability is necessary for selection to occur. Over millennia any spectrum of genetic transmission should be shifted away from the adverse and toward the helpful, depending of the demands made upon us by the environment we live in. Henry Maudsley, the first professor of psychiatry, once wrote 'In the long run it is perhaps better for the species that there is, here and there, a family stock of such constitutional instability and tendency to variation, even though variation fated to go astray, than it would be for every stock to rest in the stable equilibrium of a set adaptation to its surroundings, bee-like in busy, or sheep-like in placid routine of automatic existence.' If you develop a number of gene mutations that are considered 'unhelpful' you must have an explanation for why they persist in a significant number of the population.

The failure of natural selection argument only works as an explanation for the more severe cases of depression, which are, indeed, rare. There is an assumption that the multiple genes act additively, so it would be unlucky to inherit all of them. It is in the fat part of the bell curve that we will find most depressives, whose illness will only be triggered in response to stress, and whose illness will not be too severe or handicapping – the sort of depression which might be brought to the attention of a family doctor but not a psychiatrist. As is the nature of distribution curves, only a minority of people will fall at the extremes. Just as the recurrent severe depressive illnesses, which are seemingly not triggered by life events, are considered abnormal by most people in a given society, so the people who do not get depressed following a terrible tragedy might be considered abnormal, or 'unfeeling'.

So, this is not really an argument against the idea that depression, as experienced by the whole population, is adaptive – quite the opposite. It is simply an explanation for how the extremes of any adaptation can be perpetuated along with the adaptive middle ground.

Box 5.2 Developmental instability

The idea of 'developmental instability' also challenges the notion that depression has anything to do with natural selection. In general the model proposes that 'toxic' environmental conditions prevent us from buffering against the effects of genetic mutations. In the case of depression stressful upbringings or, let us say, viruses which invade the brain could lead to abnormal connections being made between the brain cells during early brain development. This would then make us more vulnerable to subsequent stress. However, this is not consistent with the evidence which suggests that depression has persisted for millennia because you must then explain how the same 'depression-making' mutations have persisted, and how these must have been transmitted through the generations alongside the same toxic environmental conditions that interact with them.

References

1 Buss DM. *Evolutionary psychology: the new science of the mind.* London: Allyn and Bacon; 1999.

2 Morgan E. *The scars of evolution.* London: Penguin; 1990.

3 Nesse R and Williams G. *Evolution and healing: the new science of Darwinian medicine.* London: Orion; 1996.

4 Nesse RM. The smoke detector principle; natural selection and the regulation of defensive responses. *Annals of the New York Academy of Sciences.* 2001; **935**: 75–85.

5 Buss DM, Larsen RJ, Westen D *et al.* Sex differences in jealousy: evolution, physiology, and psychology. *Psychological Science.* 1992; **3**: 251–5.

6 Fox R. *The Search for society: quest for a biosocial science and morality.* New Brunswick: Rutgers University Press; 1989.

7 Henderson S. Care-eliciting behavior in man. *Journal of Nervous Mental Disorders.* 1974; **159**: 172–81.

8 Strack S and Coyne JC. Social confirmation of dysphoria: shared and private reactions to depression. *Journal of Personality and Social Psychology.* 1983; **44**: 798–806.

9 Sacco WP and Dunn VK. Effect of actor depression on observer attributions: existence and impact of negative attributions toward the depressed. *Journal of Personality and Social Psychology.* 1990; **59**: 517–24.

10 Sacco WP, Milana S and Dunn VK. Effect of depression level and length of acquaintance on reactions of others to a request for help. *Journal of Personality and Social Psychology.* 1985; **49**:1728–37.

11 Crow TJ. Is schizophrenia the price that *Homo sapiens* pay for language? *Schizophrenia Research.* 1997; **28**: 127–141.

12 Darwin C. *The expression of the emotions in animals and man.* 3rd ed. London: Harper Collins; 1999.

13 Brown R and Lenneberg EH. A study in language and cognition. *Journal of Abnormal and Social Psychology.* 1954; **49**: 454–62.

14 Beck AT. *Cognitive therapy and the emotional disorders.* 4th ed. Madison, CT: International University Press Inc.; 1976.

15 Papadakis AA, Prince RP, Jones NP *et al.* Self-regulation, rumination, and vulnerability to depression in adolescent girls. Papadakis. *Development and Psychopathology.* 2006; **18**: 815–29.

16 Raes F, Hermans D, Williams JM *et al.* Reduced autobiographical memory specificity and rumination in predicting the course of depression. *Journal of Abnormal Psychology.* 2006; **115**: 699–704.

17 Eysenck HJ. *The structure of human personality.* London: Methuen; 1970.

18 Kuyken W, Watkins E, Holden E *et al.* Rumination in adolescents at risk for depression. *Journal of Affective Disorders.* 2006; **96**: 39–47. Epub 11 July 2006.

19 Heim C and Nemeroff CB. The role of childhood trauma in the neurobiology of mood and anxiety disorders: preclinical and clinical studies. *Biological Psychiatry.* 2001; **49**:1023–39.

20 Hinshelwood R, Robinson S and Zarate O. *Introducing Melanie Klein.* London: Icon Books; 2005.

21 Davidson RJ, Lewis DA, Alloy LB *et al.* Neural and behavioural substrates of mood and mood regulation. *Biological Psychiatry.* 2002; **52**: 478–502.

22 Dobson KS and Shaw BF. Cognitive assessment with major depressive disorders. *Cognitive Therapy and Research.* 1986;**10**: 13–29.

23 Reid AH. *The psychiatry of mental handicap.* London: Blackwell Scientific; 2005.

24 Ellinson CG. Religious involvement and subjective well-being. *Journal of Health and Social Behaviour.* 1991; **32**: 80–99.

25 French S and Joseph S. Religiosity and its association with happiness, purpose in life and self-actualisation. *Mental Health, Religion and Culture.* 1999; **2**: 117–120.

26 Jones EL. A study of traditional prayer, inner healing prayer and psychological well-being among evangelical Christians. *Dissertation Abstracts International, Section B: the Sciences and Engineering.* 1998.

What has depression ever done for us?

CHAPTER 6

Putting on the brakes

Depression stops us chasing rainbows.
Paul Gilbert[1]

Our evolutionary understanding of psychology lags far behind our understanding of physical attributes because there are no fossils of human behaviour. We would have no hesitation in attempting to give Darwinian explanations for why we have erect spines, why we have developed the skill of opposition (the ability to bring finger and thumb together), why reflex arcs have developed to ensure a quick withdrawal response to pain, or why we are so sensitive to movements in our peripheral vision. These arguments are all well established – opposition enabled us to use tools, reflex arcs clearly prevent injury, being bipedal might have made us better at hunting, and peripheral vision is important to see predators. But do we have *psychological* adaptations? And how could depression be an adaptation?

A sensible first step in creating a theory about how depression might have helped our ancestors is to consider what social conditions of today tend to provoke stress-related and depressive biological reactions in both humans and animals, given that our biology is still in the caves.

Getting detached

We know that being separated from those who love us and care for us is possibly the most potent trigger for misery that we can experience, and we have learnt that animals react to separation in depressive ways too. Separation is not only a trigger for short-term misery, anxiety and stress; it is also a well known trigger for depression.

It could be argued that the unpleasant emotions we experience in the early stages of separation motivate behaviour aimed at retrieving the missing person. All we can do as infants is cry, and hope that this triggers a nurturing response in the mother. As adults, we can be more proactive and the stress response prepares us for the possible hard struggle to be reunited. If we can retrieve our estranged loved one quickly then these negative feelings will subside, and we will almost instantly feel much happier. In future disputes with our nearest and dearest, memories of this roller-coaster ride of emotional experience might make us think twice before breaking ties with them again.

It clearly makes sense, from an evolutionary point of view, to retrieve our current caregivers (if we are infants) and lovers (if we are adults); this will maximise our survival and reproductive potential, respectively. If we fail to retrieve them it may be a long time before we find someone else to care for us or procreate with us, particularly if we live in a hostile environment.

All reactions to separation, sometimes called grief, contain a depressive phase – what the researchers of infant humans and monkeys called the 'despair phase', where the anxious yearning is replaced by sullen resentment, slowing, sadness and lack of motivation. In most people this phase continues for days or weeks before being replaced by anger and then acceptance and this is considered to be a normal process. However, in terms of symptoms, this phase of grief (or more generally what we call a 'loss adjustment') can be difficult to separate from depression, as we discussed in Chapter 4. It is no easier to appreciate just how such a prolonged state of incapacity could be useful as it is to consider the benefits of what we choose to call depression. Depressed people are unattractive and unmotivated – they lack the drive to be reunited with the estranged party that is seen in the early stages of grief. They are less hopeful of reconciliation. However, this resigned feature of the depressive phase might be the very feature that proves to be useful in the long term. Taking the long-term view is the key to understanding depression's potential to help us. The work of the hugely influential psychologist John Bowlby illustrates this.

In 1973 Bowlby published a summary of the findings of many studies which had examined the effect of separating young children (between 15 and 30 months old) from their mothers.[2] All the children had been placed in a nursery or hospital ward, with limited visiting hours, after previously enjoying close and secure attachments to their caregivers. He observed the initial stages of protest, lasting for a few days, followed by the depressive stage of despair. However, he also noted a third stage, occurring after many days or weeks of despair, which he called 'detachment'. This stage was often welcomed as a sign of recovery. It was characterised by a return of interactive behaviour – the child would start to accept the care of nurses, accept food and toys, and to smile and be sociable. In other words, the child appeared to be coming out of a depression and returning to normal. However, on the mother's return the child would no longer try to make contact with her. He would behave in a *detached* or indifferent manner to her presence, remaining remote and listlessly turning away. This sequence of reactions dovetails with the adult adjustment to loss – anxiety, depression, and then acceptance.

Thus, the depressive second stage seems to act as an instinctive means by which an initially distressing personal loss becomes acknowledged and *accepted*.[2] This is as true for adults as it is for infants, and the process seems to be unwilled. As the common adage goes, time is the healer; the process can not be speeded up, and one can not skip straight from stress to acceptance, the depressive phase needs to come in-between. Depression seems to be required in order to put on the brakes – mentally and physically. In adulthood, these reactions to separation stop us from chasing after the lover who is spurning us or the boss who is refusing to give us promotion. Depression is a counterpoint to the initial drive for reconciliation which is clearly not succeeding. It makes us give up hope, or to be more realistic about the prospect of recovering what is lost. This is true even of bereavement, because there is a fantasy that the deceased will return.

If we do not move on we become stuck. Some might call this state denial; others might call it 'pathological grief'.[3] There will usually be some added factor that makes it very difficult for the person to break away. That factor may be guilt, social isolation, ambiguous feelings towards a deceased person or a missed opportunity to say goodbye, to achieve 'closure'. The term closure was introduced in 1910 by the Gestalt school of therapy in Germany to describe the way scattered and troubling feelings can resolve themselves in coherent and stable mental patterns.[4] As Robert Fulford wrote in *The National Post* in 2001, 'Today, it means much more – coming to terms emotionally with tragedy, or rapidly ending the misery caused by grievous loss.'[5]

Depression occurs in other situations – like the failure to achieve a higher social rank. This could serve a positive fitness function in the *longer term* because, in most cases, we would be better off forming close bonds with people who are more attentive to our needs. In other words, as an infant it is important for survival to detach from unreliable caregivers and form new bonds with more constant carers.

This detachment function has a fitness advantage in adult life also. As an adult, finding a new sexual partner after being rejected by a former lover is of primary importance for the further propagation of our genes. Moreover, partners with whom we have bonded tend to provide us with assistance and protection when we are ill or otherwise compromised.

Thus, it is tempting to suggest that the primary function of depression is to achieve detachment from lost figures, but this would not be the whole story. We have learnt that depression occurs in conditions of entrapment, persistent threat and humiliating defeat, otherwise known as loss of social ranking. Let us first of all consider rank.

Social status

Status is something all humans instinctively strive for (see Box 6.1). Some people believe that depression is all about social status, or rank – that it is a way of forcing us to accept that we will not achieve our ambitions to get to the top, despite all our efforts. Again, the three stages of adjustment seem to be present: the first is the stressful fight, which becomes prolonged due to the persistent barrier to success (this is like the reaction to the mother or lover who does not return); the second is depression; the third is acceptance.

Again, experiments on primates have informed our understanding of human ways of dealing with status shifts, and have evolutionary implications. Arguably the most important research on rank carried out over the past 30 years is the work on social hierarchies in vervet monkeys by Raleigh and McGuire at the University of California.[6] It was these researchers who first introduced the term 'alpha male' to the general lexicon, describing the strongest and most competitive males at the top of the social tree. They discovered that alpha males had a higher turnover of the chemical serotonin in their brains than those at the bottom of the hierarchy. Low levels of brain serotonin are also associated with depression.

When animals aspiring to be alpha males lost their dominant positions, not only did their brain levels of serotonin plummet but they behaved in the same way as the depressed macaque monkeys described earlier – they huddled together, rocked, refused food and looked very

---

Box 6.1   The need for status

In our ancestors' environment it would have been important for us to achieve as high a status as possible within a group, irrespective of gender, because status is linked to differential reproductive success. In general, someone with a high-ranking status can enjoy better protection from enemies and predators, a greater share of the society's resources, and more access to the best mating partners.[5] Therefore, humans within any society have an instinct to compete to try to achieve the highest status that they can, even if this involves some danger. These instincts persist to the present day, but are commonly replaced by 'status symbols'.

In recent times men have often been accused of being 'too competitive'. Women, however, have never been divorced from status battles. Some societies have been matriarchal, the most familiar examples being the Amazonian warrior communities. In the modern western world women now hold high-status positions in commerce, law and political life. In more restrictive patriarchal societies women have nonetheless competed – for the man who not only looks strong and athletic but who also has resources; the ultimate basis of this struggle being that the strong and well-resourced man can provide the best protection for the pregnant woman and her offspring.

---

similar to depressed humans. These behaviours were prevented by prescribing antidepressants that raise serotonin transmission in certain parts of the brain.

In another experiment, if the alpha male was removed and another randomly chosen male was given antidepressants that male became the new alpha male.

Raleigh and McGuire's findings must be interpreted with caution because high serotonin levels are associated not only with a lack of depression, but also with aggressive behaviour. Therefore, the alpha males may have had higher levels of serotonin because they were more aggressive, and giving antidepressants may have had an effect on promotion in the hierarchy that was independent of depression.

Nevertheless, the results seem to be in keeping with all the other animal models of depression that we have looked at – the common elements being some sort of chronic stress. With other models the cause of the stress was a prolonged separation or entrapment in a threatening situation. In the case of status depression appears to be a check on unbridled (and perhaps unrealistic) ambition to get ahead. It is a process of involuntary yielding that stops those with more ambition than strength from getting drawn into a prolonged battle, with risk of injury, wasted energy and ultimate failure, perhaps even social isolation and death. The proposed benefits of depression, therefore, are that the animal does not waste energy and avoids physical harm. I propose that similar mechanisms have been inherited by humans, and that is why we see depression in ambitious businessmen who fail to get promoted. In antiquity similar goals existed – to become respected warriors, hunters or suitors.

There are additional benefits in this context too: in a potentially violent status battle the depressed person no longer looks like a threat to his opponent. We can see the depressive reaction at work in a more temporary sense during an athletics track event. The winner of the one hundred metres sprint obviously behaves very differently from the loser. The body language says everything about the contrasting emotional states. The winner is confident, energetic and walks tall. He celebrates with the crowd and may later go 'out on the town' to celebrate. The loser is hunched, hangs his head, and keeps a low profile, tending to quietly slink off home. He looks drained of energy and animation. These reactions are universal human reactions to winning or losing a contest. The defeat state experienced by the weaker adversary causes him to lose all energy and, in a physical fight, he would be forced to abandon all further attempts to beat his adversary. The attempts to look strong are replaced by 'yielding behaviour' – the defeated will make himself small, keep still, and show anguish.[7] As aggression seems to be intimately linked to threat, the fight does not normally continue.

So, depression is a *prolonged* defeat state arising in circumstances in which we have not engaged in yielding behaviour at the appropriate time, despite being met with stronger forces. It is arguably necessary not only for putting on the brakes, but to move us towards acceptance, like the depressive reactions to separation. If we have unrealistic expectations, or have false information, or if we are trying to please two people at once we might fail to yield at an early stage. Depression forces us to reassess the situation when no progress is being made and helps us to reconsider whether we can achieve the status we crave, or whether we have the right strategy for achieving it. In other words, following re-assessment of internal and external factors, and acceptance of our previous failings, we might then be in a better position to compete more successfully. This would clearly be adaptive in the long term. It seems that every argument for depression's adaptiveness is about weighing up the short-term pain and longer-term gain.

Not all writers on the evolutionary origins of depression agree with this interpretation of depression and status, however. It has been proposed, for example, that depression evolved for the good of the group: to reduce conflict and to let people know their place.[8] In other words, if people try to get above their station and become socially mobile, depression will come along and send them down again. It is proposed that this allows for stratification and order, given that people have different levels of energy, drive, talent and skill. However, this 'social homeostasis' idea is a form of group selection, and group selection has been largely discredited.[9] Individual benefits are more important in evolutionary terms than group benefits. If depression had caused sufferers to sink to lower ranks, never to compete again, those in the lower ranks would have been selected out in favour of the stronger members of the species. Over the course of millennia, depression would have bowed out of the gene pool. Clearly this has not occurred. Depression has persisted. There are other objections too. Firstly, depression is an episodic, or self-limiting, condition. Secondly, people in lower ranks of society, in terms of economic wealth, are not necessarily depressed. In many cases they can be happier than those who are more competitive. Finally, research has told us that it is humiliating defeat that triggers depression, not being in a lower rank per se. The disparity between reality and expectation is important.

It is also true that in any social hierarchy there are many different domains in which one may compete. Failing in one domain does not preclude succeeding in another. Hence depression may cause someone to bow out of competing in one domain (like doctor, healer or warrior), only to return to the fight in another competitive arena (like entertainer, builder or hunter). This would be helpful for the group but more importantly, in evolutionary terms, it would help to promote the long-term success of the individual. Recent research contradicts the idea that people who have experienced depressed function worse as a result. Some studies suggest that depression might improve occupational functioning.[10,11] This may have come about as a result of reassessment and trying a different strategy. We will discuss how depression might aid reassessment in the next chapter.

Chronic stress and frustrated goals

We have looked at two plausible theories of depression's ultimate function; detachment from those who do not love or care for us, and yielding against stronger adversaries in order to abandon unrealistic goals or rethink the strategy for achieving success.

However, although plausible, both of these theories overlook Seligman's findings on learned helplessness, which dovetail with the evidence that entrapment in situations of threat also provokes depression in humans.[12] How is this helpful?

The quick answer to this is that it isn't, but if you are trapped in a situation of inescapable stress beyond your control you are probably not going to survive long anyway. Perhaps depression kicks in instinctively, because it has evolved to be triggered by chronic stress, whatever the cause, in order to conserve precious energy and focus the mind on solutions. In some cases, a solution can be found, because the entrapment is virtual not literal. There may be an internal barrier to escape – the fear of the alternative situation, or fear of the unknown. If the stress has been chronic so has the fear of escape, and this is because the solution needed to escape is drastic – perhaps requiring us to walk out of a town, country, family, relationship or a career. It could be we can only take such radical steps if faced with the grim reality of depression.

The idea that persisting stress is a common pathway to depression makes sense if we go back to thinking about the triggers in the modern day. So, a bereavement that leads to isolation and poverty for the person left behind will be more 'depressogenic' (depression generating) than a bereavement that occurs in the context of social and financial security. A divorce is more likely to lead to depression if there is ensuing acrimony between the divorcees, and protracted custody battles. Losing one's job might not lead to depression if one found the job very stressful, but depression will be more likely if one subsequently loses one's house, wife and the respect of friends. These problems have long-term implications. The chronic difficulties that follow the event are often crucial in the genesis of depression, not just the acute event itself. Events with long-term threat will tend to be events with long-term negative consequences.

Also, a person who experiences an adverse life event against a background of ongoing life difficulties will be more prone to experiencing depression than someone who perceives that he is sailing along without apparent problems. In other words, one negative life event can be the 'straw that breaks the camel's back'. We have learnt that adverse life events are more likely to trigger depression in women who have three or more children under the age of fourteen to look after in the home. Also, it has been shown that a match between ongoing difficulties and events is more likely to lead to depression – a phenomenon sometimes called 'contextual threat'.[13] For example, a son may be jailed against a background of ongoing discord with his mother. The mother is vulnerable to developing depression in this situation. However, if she had formerly enjoyed positive relations with her child she would have been less vulnerable.

So, much of the evidence from the modern world suggests that adult depression is a non-specific reaction to any stress that has been going on for a long time.

Let us consider, therefore, what triggers stress from an evolutionary point of view. Can evolutionary psychology provide a unifying theme? In evolution there is one overriding law – and that is to behave in such a way that will maximise our fitness. Provided we are healthy and conscious we will never stop striving to reach goals that are important for the perpetuation of our genes. There are six main types of goal, which we can call archetypal needs:

- *sustenance* the need to obtain food and drink
- *personal resources* athleticism, good health, shelter
- *social resources* being loved and respected by others who might help and protect us
- *status/rank* obtaining the highest possible status within the group
- *reproductive success* finding a partner and procreating
- *children* protecting the vessels of our genes and raising them.

The fight for these goals is not necessarily conscious, and modern life is so awash with abstractions that we fail to realise what are fundamental needs really are. Nevertheless we are simple organisms at heart – vessels for propagating our genes, and slaves to the instincts to preserve them.[14] Stress is what we feel when any effort to achieve these goals is frustrated. It is always accompanied by negative mood, which is there to motivate us to try harder, at least initially.

Maslow's hierarchy of archetypal needs argues that some needs are more important than others because they have a more direct impact on the propagation of our genes (see Figure 6.1).[15] So, for example, if we do not obtain shelter and security we will not survive for long enough to procreate. If we do not belong to a social group we may lack the stability to maintain a sexual relationship, and so on. The needs must be met in the right order.

People who strive for occupational success in the modern world while neglecting a marriage at home are frustrating two archetypal intents at the same time: achieving a higher rank will lead to a greater share of resources, better security and, possibly, a better chance of procreating, but if your wife leaves you during the struggle, the status battle will be rendered meaningless from the point of view of archetypal needs.

The negative emotional state that we develop in the early stages of goal frustration – of sadness, anger, guilt, jealousy or anxiety (the type of emotion depends on the context) – drives us harder toward achieving the goal. We also develop a stress response which physiologically

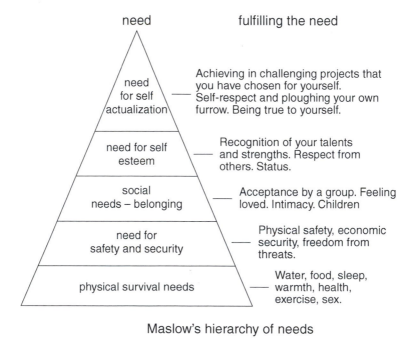

Maslow's hierarchy of needs

Figure 6.1 A hierarchy of archetypal needs (adapted from Maslow)

prepares us for expending greater effort in the face of obstacles. I will call this combination of stress response and negative emotion the 'goal frustration state'.

It follows that depression will occur if this goal frustration state becomes protracted. Normally we resolve stressful situations quickly – either by finding a way round an obstacle, or by choosing a different direction – but sometimes we plough on, regardless of the fact that there is little movement toward the goal. This denial can arise for either internal or external reasons, which we will explore in the next chapter (see Figure 6.2).

Depression forces us to give up in these situations. Once depression has been triggered it puts the brakes on. Further effort toward achieving the elusive goal becomes very difficult and the struggle is finally abandoned.

It seems that our bodies are designed to cope with acute stress, but the long term health consequences of protracted stress are seen in animals and man: peptic ulcer disease, psoriasis, heart disease, cancer, stroke and, ultimately, death. Consistently high stress hormones lead to what the early animal researchers called 'adrenal exhaustion'.

So, depression, although linked to health problems (for reasons we discussed in the previous chapter), may in fact curtail much worse health consequences by removing us from the situation that is causing protracted stress. In other words, even though depression is subjectively unpleasant, and feels like a stressful experience in itself, it may actually represent an important withdrawal mechanism. And also, converse as it may seem, depression has long been linked to the idea of energy conservation; this is in spite of the fact that sufferers often suffer insomnia and rarely feel rested. From an evolutionary point of view, the conservation of energy would have been very important to our ancestors due to their more limited access to food, water and secure lodging.

A human hibernation

Judging by external appearances depression seems well designed to cause us to withdraw from stressful, futile activity and conserve energy. All the psychic and bodily functions are slowed down. There is a slowing of mentation (thought processes), speech, voluntary movement (what psychiatrists call 'psychomotor retardation') and a slowing of the automatic regulation of bodily function, like bowel

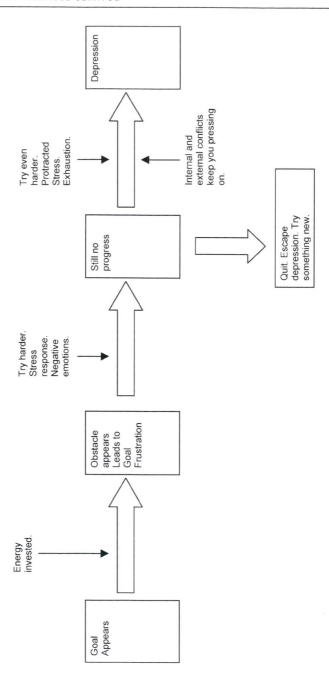

Figure 6.2 Goal frustration and depression

movements. There is a tendency towards lethargy and inactivity, otherwise known as torpor.

The torpor associated with human depression has led some authors to suggest that it is equivalent to the state of hibernation seen in animals such as bears.[16] Intriguingly, antidepressants have been shown to reduce the amount of torpor in hibernating golden hamsters.[17] Furthermore lithium, a drug used to prevent recurrent episodes of depression in humans, has also been shown to prevent hibernation in Turkish hamsters.[18] Also, as in the case of a hibernating mammal, depression is associated with a reduction in appetite. In the face of seriously depleted resources, due to a protracted and futile expenditure of energy, this symptom should be beneficial.

Seasonal affective disorder (SAD) is a particular form of depression that consistently and exclusively occurs during the winter months. For this reason it is often known as winter depression.[19] SAD probably has different evolutionary origins from generic depression but it is relevant to any discussion of its conservation–withdrawal function. It has often been regarded as a form of energy conservation – a kind of human hibernation. There are grounds for regarding SAD as a special type of depression for two reasons. First, rather than a reaction to difficulties or events, SAD is believed to occur due to a relative lack of sunlight. Second, the symptoms are different: SAD is characterised by too much sleep rather than too little sleep, and is typically associated with carbohydrate craving, and weight gain, rather than a reduction in appetite.

SAD is a feature of people living in northern latitudes, where the winters are long, cold and dark. Both of the typical SAD symptoms described above could be regarded as adaptive to such conditions. Historically, it was common for humans to build up their fat stores before winter, when meat was still relatively plentiful. During winter, when food was scarce, and hunting and gathering were difficult, it would have made sense to conserve one's energy by sleeping, and to eat energy-rich food when it was available. Carbohydrates are a readily utilisable source of energy. They are more easily digested than fat, and the energy is released to the body more quickly: when one's body is running slowly, substances that are more readily digested will be preferred. Some hibernating animals will suffer indigestion if they are fed with foods rich in fat and protein, although they stock up on fat rich foods prior to hibernation.

The carbohydrate preference, weight gain and the increased need for sleep seen in SAD, or atypical depression, are a better match with the physiological changes seen in hibernating animals than the insomnia and weight loss seen in more typical depression. The reduced reproductive drives seen in both SAD and hibernating animals lend further support to the human hibernation idea. A lack of reproduction in the winter months is an important way of characterising a species as a hibernator; of SAD patients, 69 per cent report reduced libido.[20,21]

However, there is a wide variety of hibernating strategies in the animal kingdom. Only some hibernating animals (like the golden hamster) hibernate in response to changes in day length, and not all animals have a period of torpor that corresponds to the winter months. Some hibernating animals have biannual periods of torpor; others do not demonstrate reduced activity at all, but merely a 'fattening' period prior to winter. Whether SAD represents a subtle form of light-sensitive hibernation like that seen in golden hamsters or bears is debatable, and this question is in fact a distraction from the main point: SAD could well be a mechanism for conserving energy during the winter months in lineages whose distant ancestors lived in particularly harsh winter conditions. The generic depressive illness may well represent a similar conservation strategy, but one that occurs after internal and external resources have been pushed to the limit.

There are some challenges to the conservation–withdrawal idea. As I stated above, people who are depressed rarely *feel* rested. Some cases of depression are characterised by restlessness. Also, depressed people do not enjoy restful sleep. One would have thought that a mechanism designed to conserve energy would lead to improvements in sleep patterns, whereas depressed people actually experience less deep (slow-wave) sleep than non-depressed people.[22] Characteristically when they rise in the morning they do not feel refreshed. The hibernation analogy breaks down here: hibernating animals sleep more deeply (have more slow-wave sleep) than non-hibernators. Furthermore, evidence of the presence of elevated cortisol (the stress hormone) in at least a large proportion of people with depression, and most people with severe psychotic depression, further weakens the conservation hypothesis.[23]

However, the actual role of cortisol in the body remains to be clarified, and its relationship to stress-related physical harm or exhaustion is still unclear. Also, an adaptation does not have to be comfortable to the individual in order to be adaptive. Our coughing and vomiting reactions are not pleasant, but they are helpful – they are defences against noxious substances threatening to invade our bodies.Perhaps depression is still a useful defence, even if it is not subjectively restful or pleasant. It is possible that being depressed is less harmful to the body, and, crucially, less costly in resources, than striving for an unobtainable goal over a long period of time.

The power of the group

So, we have a unifying theory of how depression might work in an adaptive way:

1   it takes us out of chronically stressful situations or states of mind (so we avoid injury, the physical complications of chronic stress, and conserve energy)
2   it makes us reassess, and then
3   we re-enter society with a new perspective.

However, so far we have not addressed how our depressed ancestors could have coped in the short term until the depression lifted. Were they not more prone to attack from enemies and predators in their defeated, sluggish and lethargic state? Were they not less capable of hunting or foraging for food? The potential threat to survival seems clear.

However, a review of what we have just discussed makes us realise that the immobile and withdrawn state reduces the risk of attack. It is probable that depressed people would have withdrawn from situations where they might have been preyed upon (in the same way that they tend to withdraw from social contact in the modern environment), and their yielding behaviour would have reduced the outward appearance of threat. The slowed up state demands less energy and hence the need for sustenance is reduced.

More contentiously, our depressed ancestors might have enjoyed increased support from close members of their own community to help them through the worst of the blues. Archaeological evidence suggests that until about 40,000 years ago we lived in tight knit hunter–gatherer communities consisting of only about 40 to 50 people.[24] This is how we have lived for 99.5 per cent of our evolutionary history. The basic state of our ancestral society included between six and ten adult males, about twice as many child-bearing females, and about 20 juveniles and infants. These intimate and close-knit groups shared the same values, mores, and codes of conduct, including marriage and mourning, reinforced by rituals and religious beliefs. There would have been regular contact between different groups. Gifts, greetings, feasts and other ceremonies would have helped to keep the peace (see Box 6.2).

Box 6.2 Why have we always been such social animals?
Among the different social systems within a group, the most clearly identified in most primates and humans are the nurturing role of the mother, the bond developed between mother and infant (so that the infant keeps in close proximity), the heterosexual bonding system and the paternal system (whereby the strong male wards off predators and protects women and children).[25] Human infants are poor at defending themselves from attack and they can not sustain themselves. A human child can not forage or hunt or run from predators until about the age of seven.[26] Being in a group is important for maintaining the family unit and nurturing and protecting our offspring.

However, there are other evolutionary explanations for the instinctive group behaviour of humans. Hunting in groups, for example, was more efficient and effective than hunting alone. As a result, each individual enjoyed access to more food within a group than he would have done if he had chosen to be a lone wolf. Also, a division of labour could occur within a group so that individual skills could be maximally exploited. Groups could better protect themselves from natural predators, could build stronger shelters, and could more effectively fight off other competing humans. Finally, an individual within a group could be protected when he was ill or infirm, just as the helpless infant could be protected. The social conditions of the ancestral hunter (living in a group of 50 people) may have represented the best compromise between the advantages and costs of living with a number of other humans. Supportive relationships might not have developed so readily in larger groups. Rival groups might have started to develop. A larger group might have been less efficient at fairly allocating resources.

Since depression was first delineated as a specific disorder by Kraepelin, the father of modern European psychiatry, we have known that it is typically self-limiting, or episodic, lasting for weeks or months.[27]

Spontaneous remission occurs in most cases. Therefore, in the majority of cases, the person afflicted with depression will eventually be able to perform a useful function within the wider society. It makes sense, for the welfare of the group, that he be patiently nursed back to recovery. If the depressed individual is ejected, the effectiveness and efficiency of the group is diminished. As long as someone adopts a valid sick role it is arguably a human instinct to provide care and support, because the favour will be returned when we are in trouble, and because being a member of a group of well-functioning adults will improve the fitness of that member.

But is depression a special case of illness in this regard? Perhaps, rather than stimulating caring instincts in people, depression repels potential carers. Depressed people can be very difficult to help. They are poor company – hopeless, depressing, and occasionally irritable or hostile. Sometimes they even reject help, which is a violation of the 'sick role'.[28] We resent people who are not grateful when we try to help them. The depressed person often responds to help by feeling guilty, without appreciating that the help will be ultimately beneficial. He may be so hopeless that he believes that all help is futile. A lot of patience is required in dealing with a depressed person, and patience requires a good deal of understanding. The degree to which depressed people are difficult to like probably depends on the prevailing attitudes of the community, and memories of how the depressed person behaved when he was well. The closer you are to someone, the more likely it is that you will tolerate their depressive behaviour and do everything in your power to ensure that recovery comes swiftly.

There is evidence accrued since the early experimental psychology studies that, in general, depressed people do indeed engender the caring role in close community members such as close friends, certain family members or partners, without there being a request for 'reciprocal help'.[29] This is in spite of the difficult behaviour that some depressed people demonstrate. However, as we learnt in the last chapter, the jury is still out on this topic – many people have demonstrated that depression is, by its very nature, antisocial, and that depressed people are avoided by other members of their community, even if it is close knit. Depressed people are criticised and shunned, especially if they remain depressed for a year or more. As empathic creatures we are easily infected by the melancholy of others, and hence we seek to avoid protracted contact with depressed people. Our dislike of depressed people is probably matched by the depressed person's dislike of social contact. The truly depressed individual desires isolation, and this feature of depression might well have evolved to fit with the needs of the community; the depressive feels that sociability requires too much effort and lacks the spark that people find attractive.

This has prompted evolutionary psychologists to search for another theory, which is about the *delayed* advantages of getting depressed within a close-knit community, in terms of long-term influence on the social group, or increased 'social navigation'.[30] Whether depression leads to increased help in the short term or not, in the longer term the depressed person may unwittingly extort extra help from others that was lacking in the past. For example, Ed Hagen's 'strike hypothesis' proposes that clinical depression helps the depressive to prompt more generous behaviour from a formerly exploitative community member or partner.[31] In the short term, someone who goes on strike will forego some pay and may be derided by many people, including the employer, some colleagues, possibly the press, and possibly the general public. Similarly, depression can have a very negative effect on others, often attracting criticism and disdain. Depression imposes enormous costs – on the sufferer, his family and friends, the local community and society in general. Even people who are close to the sufferer may not understand his or her behaviour, finding it unsettling and pulling away, leaving him or her to cope in isolation.

However, returning to the strike analogy, *in the longer term* a person who is on strike may later achieve a pay deal that is fair given his level of skills and training, because ultimately his skills and training are needed by management. Similarly, the person who is 'on strike' with depression in a close, interdependent community can deprive the community in which he lives, because his input is needed. In antiquity we would have lived in such small groups that the sense of loss over a member 'striking' would have been acute – he or she would have been sorely missed. These days, when we have looser ties to each other, we might not be missed so much. However, that is not the fault of depression; it is the fault of changes in society, an example of how depression may have become less adaptive over time because there is a difference between the social conditions of today and those in which it originally evolved.

In the case of a properly supportive community, depression should be a short-term pain for longer-term gain. If you become depressed this can hurt others more than it hurts you, and therefore those who are close to you will normally do their best to understand what caused your depression and help you to remedy the situation and move forward. This even extends, in 'bargaining theory', to suicidal gestures.[32] Suicidal ideas and suicide attempts greatly outnumber successful suicides, and they may be a method of negotiating a better deal in life. Depression may even prompt problem-solving suggestions from friends and family, particularly with regard to social problems. There is an important reservation about the strike hypothesis, however: depression can recur, especially in people who do not, or cannot, deal with their issues. Only research carried out over many years could accurately reveal whether the increased awareness of an individual's needs, which might be extorted by depression, would wane with every subsequent episode. A 'boy who cried wolf' phenomenon could occur, with each successive cry for help being met with an increasingly dismissive or cynical response from the inured community. However, anthropological studies in Uganda reveal that individuals with recurrent depression are not shunned, but rather they are regarded as in need of help.[33]

The prevalence of depression in Uganda, a country affected by a violent political history, an HIV epidemic and the re-emergence of TB, is estimated to be 10 to 25 per cent.[34,35] A pilot study carried out in a village in the Buganda region, offered insightful vignettes about the understanding of depressed people, and the treatment of them.[33] Depression is conceptualised as a problem of 'thinking too much', and is otherwise known as the 'Illness of thoughts'. The impact is that the afflicted individual can not enjoy the company of others and withdraws – 'Too many thoughts detach you from people. You will be there. You don't want anybody to call you. You see someone laughing and you think they are laughing at you'. This is either understood as a result of the clan – an inherited condition, or as a result of the stresses of life. The 'illness of thoughts' is clearly recognised as a condition that requires compassion and help from the community and, if necessary, the assistance of a traditional healer. It is believed that there is no medication that can help, because there is no medication for thoughts. Both men and women identified illness of a close relative and death of a spouse to be important cases, but worries about money were also important. Gender specific considerations were infidelity of the male partner in women, and for a man, being left to look after his children alone. Biological explanations included HIV (organic depression due to HIV virus invading the brain is recognised) and the influence of coming from a particular clan (inheritance). Overall, however, depression was thought to come about for social and economic reasons, including a history of child abuse.

Lay help from family, close friends, experienced elders and religious leaders was identified as an important source of help for the 'illness of thoughts'. Touchingly, there was an awareness of the challenges involved in trying to help someone who shuns social contact which revealed a sympathetic understanding of the condition. Although there was evidence of stigma attached to other psychiatric conditions like mania, there was no evidence that depressed individuals were derided or deliberately excluded.

In his book *Malignant Sadness* the noted biologist Lewis Wolpert also writes on the observations of a western psychiatrist during his visit to a rural village in Uganda.[36] Depression was recognised by the symptoms of tiredness and unwillingness to work. The rest of the community made no comment on the sufferers' withdrawal from work: it was an accepted part of the life of the community. The withdrawal from the normal role was not regarded as an individual choice, which might be open to some criticism, but as an end result for some people of the interdependent way of life.

So, there is evidence that depression may indeed trigger a caring response in more traditional communities, and extort concessions with regard to normal responsibilities. Such social sanctions may allow the affected individual to embark on an important solitary journey of self-discovery. Legends, myths, tribal beliefs, and almost every religion repeat the universal theme of solitary exploration in search of personal growth. Buddha went into solitude before he achieved enlightenment; Jesus went into the desert for 40 days and 40 nights to fast and pray; Greek mythical heroes met with great tests of endurance and will in order to gain a reward: Demeter had to descend to rescue Persephone from Hades, the God of the Underworld. Psyche's descent was a prelude to her reunion with Eros. There is an ancient promise wrapped up in all these stories that a descent into the dark will nourish and bring insight, that suffering now will bring rewards later. They represent rites of passage toward enlightenment.

It is notable that Freudian psychoanalysis also contains the theme of the process of descent and re-emergence: therapy involves delving into the dark unconscious to reclaim early memories, feelings and thoughts that are painful and are therefore repressed.[37] The emergence of depressive symptoms through therapy is not unexpected, and it is traditionally regarded as a component of the healing process.[38]

Jung, Freud's contemporary, was aware of the universality of the solitary journey in his description of the archetypes contained within all human stories; these included the Hero, the Shadow and Individuation.[39] The Hero is self-explanatory – we all fantasise about being the hero of any community – we want to be loved and admired. This is one of our archetypal needs, perhaps linked with our desires for belonging, protection and status, which impact on survival and reproductive success. The Shadow is the unacknowledged part of us that is potentially destructive. It is the 'dark side' that we all share. Our solitary journeys of self-discovery are all about drawing on the dark side in positive way. The darkness brings some insights – the gold in the shadow. The concept of Individuation is about finding one's own reason for being on the earth, which might involve addressing long-repressed intellectual or spiritual needs. Although this need for individuation is particularly acute in mid-life, the process is circular and lifelong – occurring in infancy, adolescence, young adulthood, and so on. Hence the need for the solitary journey to manage life's transitions.

Some solitary journeys have become formalised into ceremonies – like the 'walkabout' of the Australian aborigines or the 'vision quest' of the native North Americans. These ceremonies are a sanctioned form of 'time out' from one's usual responsibilities within a social group. They are generally regarded as beneficial opportunities for resolving life's transitions, crises, losses, problems of stagnation and depression through introspection and communing with nature.[40] Other reasons for embarking on such a journey include seeking a deeper commitment to live life passionately, to be more open and vulnerable to love, to enhance one's creative expression and to be of greater service to one's people and community. Taking the vision quest as an example, this structured, archetypal process leads to a state of rebirth, renewal and empowerment through four main phases.[41,42]

1 *Severance* Withdrawing from the old way of living and readying oneself for the unknown; committing to a solitary journey.
2 *Purification* A time of mental, emotional and physical letting go where you enter a time of introspection into your life, relationships, difficulties and emotional suffering. The known life dies and is replaced by the cry for a new vision for life.
3 *Threshold* The heart of the vision quest. This is the time when you

venture alone into solitude, fasting and praying for a vision. This should lead to a renewed sense of self acceptance, power, peace, joy, inner strength and compassion.

4　*Reincorporation* The return to the community to share and discuss the fruits of the quest. It is also a time to begin integrating the vision you have brought back into the community.

It is apparent that the stages of the vision quest are similar to the functions we have proposed for depression itself – removal from the existing situation, introspection, problem solving, the development of a new perspective and reintegrating this with the social group upon recovery. Depression has come about due to a frustration of archetypal needs, and communing with nature in total isolation might help to remind us what those needs are – the fundamental needs that will determine our happiness, our usefulness, and, ultimately, our reproductive success.

It seems that a fundamental function for depression is the facilitation of a radical personal reassessment, a re-examination of the sufferer's fundamental needs that have hitherto been denied. One is reminded of the poem *Not Waving but Drowning* by Stevie Smith.[43] Perhaps it is better for us to be depressed, moving slowly but thoughtfully, than to be constantly out of our depth, frantically treading water until we drown. We will explore how depression might facilitate this process in more detail in the next chapter.

References

1　Gilbert P. *Overcoming Depression*. London: Constable Robinson; 2000.

2　Bowlby J. *Attachment and loss. Vol. 2. Separation: anxiety and anger*. London: Hogarth Press and the Institute of Psychoanalysis; 1973.

3　Parkes CM. *Bereavement: studies of grief in adult life*. 3rd ed. London: Penguin; 1998.

4　Perls FS. *In and out the garbage pail*. Lafayette, California: Real People Press; 1969.

5　Fulford R. *The strange popularity of the word 'closure'*. The National Post, 10 November, 2001.

6　Raleigh M and McGuire M. Serotonin in vervet monkeys. *Brain Research*. 1991; **559**: 181–90.

7　Price J. The adaptive function of mood change. *British Journal of Medical Psychology*. 1998; **71**: 465–77.

8 Stevens A and Price J. *Evolutionary psychiatry: a new beginning.* London: Routledge; 2000.

9 Barkow K, Maier W, Ustun TB *et al.* Risk factors for depression at 12-month follow-up in adult primary health care patients with major depression: an international prospective study. *Journal of Affective Disorders.* 2003; **76**: 157–69.

10 Williams GC. *Adaptation and Natural Selection.* Princeton, N.J: Princeton University Press; 1966.

11 Buist-Bouwman MA, Ormel J, de Graaf R *et al.* Functioning after a major depressive episode: complete or incomplete recovery? *Journal of Affective Disorders.* 2004; **82**: 363–71.

12 Seligman ME. Learned helplessness. *Annual Review of Medicine.* 1972; **23**:407–12.

13 Brown GW and Harris TO. Stressor, vulnerability and depression: a question of replication. *Psychological Medicine.* 1986; **16**: 739–44.

14 Dawkins R. *The selfish gene.* Oxford: Oxford University Press; 1989.

15 Maslow AH. *Motivation and personality.* New York: Harper and Row; 1954.

16 Tsiouris JA. Metabolic depression in hibernation and major depression: an explanatory theory and an animal model of depression. *Medical Hypotheses.* 2005; **65**: 829–40.

17 Zvolsky P, Jansky L, Vyskocilova J *et al.* Effects of psychotropic drugs on hamster hibernation: pilot study. *Progress in Neuro-psychopharmacology.* 1981; **5**: 599–602.

18 Giedke H and Pohl H. Lithium suppresses hibernation in the Turkish hamster. *Experentia.* 1985; **41**: 1391–2.

19 Rosenthal N. *Winter Blues.* New York: Guilford; 1993.

20 Kayser C. The intervention of external and internal factors in the determinism of the hibernation of mammals. *Archives des Sciences Physiologiques.* 1961; **15**: 377–420.

21 Rosenthal NE, Sack DA, Gillin JC *et al.* Seasonal affective disorder: a description of the syndrome and preliminary findings with light therapy. *Archives of General Psychiatry.* 1984; **41**:72–80.

22 Benca RM, Obermeyer WH, Thisted RA *et al.* Sleep and psychiatric disorders: a meta-analysis. *Archives of General Psychiatry.* 1992; **49**: 651–68.

23 Dinan TG. Psychoneuroendocrinology of mood disorders. *Current Opinion in Psychiatry.* 2001; **14**: 51–5.

24 Fox R. *The Search for Society: quest for a biosocial science and morality.* London: Rutgers University Press; 1989.

25 Harlow HF and Harlow MK. The affectional systems. In: A. M. Schrier, H. F. Harlow and F. Stollnitz (Eds.). *Behavior of nonhuman primates*. New York: Academic Press; 1965.

26 Buss DM. *Evolutionary psychology: the new science of the mind*. London: Allyn and Bacon; 1999.

27 Kraepelin E. *Psychiatric: Ein Lehrbuch*. Bristol: Thoemmes Press; 2002.

28 Cockerham W. *Medical sociology*. 8th ed. Prentice Hall; 2001.

29 Lewis AJ. Melancholia: a clinical survey of depressive states. *Journal of Mental Science*. 1934; **80**: 1–43.

30 Watson PJ and Andrews P. Toward a revised evolutionary adaptionist analysis of depression: the social navigation hypothesis. *Affect Disorders*. 2002; **72**: 1–14.

31 Hagen EH. The functions of postpartum depression. *Evolution and Human Behavior*. 1999; **20**: 325–59.

32 Hagen EH. The bargaining model of depression. In: P. Hammerstein (Ed). *Genetic and cultural evolution of cooperation*. Cambridge MA: MIT Press; 2003, p. 95–123.

33 Okello ES and Ekblad S. Lay concepts of depression among the Baganda of Uganda: a pilot study. *Transcultural Psychiatry*. 2006;**43**: 287–313.

34 German GA. Mental health in Africa: I. The extent of mental health problems in Africa today. An update of epidemiological knowledge. *British Journal of Psychiatry*. 1987;**151**: 435–9.

35 Orley J and Wing JK. Psychiatric disorders in two African villages. *Archives of General Psychiatry*. 1979; **36**: 513–20.

36 Wolpert L. *Malignant sadness: the anatomy of depression*. London: Faber and Faber; 2001.

37 Freud S. *Introductory lectures on psychoanalysis*. London: Penguin Books; 1991.

38 Greenberg LS and Pascual-Leone A. Emotion in psychotherapy: a practice-friendly research review. *Journal of Clinical Psychology*. 2006; **62**: 611–30.

39 Casement A. *Carl Gustav Jung*. London: SAGE; 2001.

40 Plotkin B. *Soulcraft: crossing into the mysteries of nature and psyche*. Novato, CA: New World Library; 2003.

41 Foster S. *The book of the vision quest*. Wichita, KS: Fireside; 1989.

42 Brown JE. *The sacred pipe: Black Elk's account of the seven rites of the Oglala Sioux*. Oklahoma: University of Oklahoma Press; 2003.

43 Smith S. *Selected poems*. London: Penguin Books; 2002.

CHAPTER 7

Taking stock (the vision quest)

Before we can try to understand the function of sadness, grief and depression in the process of self-discovery we first of all need to understand the internal and external reasons why humans would persist in a behaviour which is causing stress without a pay off. The film *Magnolia*, is a long but beautiful cinematic work consisting of the winding narratives of loosely connected people, all carrying painful emotional issues. It offers hope towards the end of the film as the characters start to confront the issues which have hitherto sent them in the wrong direction, and caused suffering, not only in themselves but in others. In this chapter we will explore how depression could help us to 'wise up' in this way.[1]

Struggling on in spite of failure: the causes of chronic stress

Reason one: Ignorance

It has been said that an ignorant man is always a slave. In the film *Jean de Florette*, a young man of the title inherits a farm and trades his life in the city for the idyll of rural France.[2] However, he is ignorant of the hidden animosity felt towards him by a neighbouring farmer Cesar, who had hoped to buy the land himself for a lower price. Cesar stops the natural spring that had been irrigating the land. Unaware of this, Jean battles hard to make the farm work, and blames his own lack of experience when the crops fail. Still, unaware of the lack of irrigation, he keeps trying to make the farm viable, but despite the stress and hardship, there is no reward for his efforts. He dies in an accident while frantically struggling to cultivate the barren land he thinks will eventually provide him and his family with a living.

Consistent with what we know about the triggers for depression, this humiliating failure was driving him towards depression. We do not know what the outcome might have been if he had not died prematurely, but if he had become depressed the venture would surely have been abandoned. He would have been forced to consider another life somewhere else, even if this would have meant starting from nothing. Unknown to him, this would have been the best policy, because poorly irrigated land will never yield a healthy crop.

(Following Jean's death, the neighbour buys the land at a reduced price, and unblocks the spring. The real tragedy, however, is revealed in the sequel, *Manon des Sources*, when the new owner of the farm realises that the man whose death was linked to his selfish intervention was, in fact, his estranged son).[3]

Also, consider the case of a husband who, due to his own insecurities, did not want his wife to work because he was afraid that she would meet attractive men. He was unable to admit this to her, but instead repeatedly criticised her work performance. She loved him but, because she did not understand the true motives behind his behaviour, she spent even more time at work and aggravated him further. The ensuing protracted conflict caused her to become depressed to the point where she was no longer able to work. The depression might have been prevented if the woman concerned had decided to leave her husband because of his behaviour, or if she had learnt about his insecurities and had then had the opportunity to address them.

Reason two: High moral scruples

This is not a plea to behave immorally; there are times when persistent adherence to higher principles or moral scruples will be in direct conflict with our fundamental needs. Socrates took on the democracy and prevailing culture of Athens rather than renounce his controversial views. Milton challenged the monarchy. Darwin challenged the church. Although these individuals carved out a place in history they also neglected their own fundamental needs as human beings. It has been suggested that all of these famous people suffered from depression as a consequence of their persistence in fighting against mightier forces. This is a noble sacrifice that some of us choose to make – and the freedom to make this choice is arguably what makes us human. Sometimes the choice is made for us due to the weight of expectation of those who rely on our leadership; sometimes greatness is forced upon us. However, we must not be surprised if our grand gestures eventually lead to depression.

Consider an example that may be closer to home, and which was originally published as a case study by the psychiatrist Jonathon Price.[4] A man failed to join his work colleagues in a dishonest plan which was designed to benefit them all financially. Each colleague was supposed to take sick leave, whether or not they were ill, so that the others could claim overtime. As a result of failing to go along with this plan, due to adherence to his higher moral scruples, the man was ostracised and punished by his colleagues, to the point where he became depressed as a consequence. Fitting in to a peer group is an archetypal need, albeit an unconscious one. However, our victim in this situation ignored that need, suffered chronic stress, and paid the price. If he had left the job voluntarily, and perhaps found a more honest working environment elsewhere, he might have prevented the onset of depression. In the end depression gave him no choice but to leave work.

Reason three: Trying to please someone else rather than ourselves

The third case in which our goals are in conflict with our needs is when pressure is being exerted by a third party. Our own goals may be frustrated in order to satisfy someone else's goals. For example, our parents may push us into a career that does not satisfy our needs, and then threaten to cut off support if we do not continue in this line of work. Sometimes we might try to please two people at the same time. We may have such strong ties to both people that we cannot avoid an internal conflict. Consider another case published by Jonathon Price, where a wife wanted to please both her husband and her mother.[4] Her husband wanted her to be at home on Saturdays, but she was unable to comply with his wishes because her mother insisted that she do chores for her on that day. She eventually became depressed because, over many months, she was unable to de-escalate the conflict with her husband. Her depression only remitted when her mother died. If the wife had stood up to her mother, or perhaps been firmer with her partner, the depression might have been avoided. According to Ed Hagen's strike hypothesis, her depression should have alerted either her mother or her husband to her plight, although it seems that only death could remedy this particular situation.[5]

Reason four: Unrealistic expectations arising from childhood

Albert Einstein once said to a protégé 'Don't try to be a man of success. Try to be man of value'.[6] His words suggest that we should not chase after status and fame for their own sake; rather we should do the best we can to achieve something important, to make in some way a significant contribution to others. Status and fame may then follow, but chasing after them at the expense of being part of a community (an archetypal need) could lead to ruin, especially as there will always be someone who has higher status and is more famous than you.

However, even if we focus more on achievement and less on fame and fortune, it is still important to recognise the difference between dreams and expectations.

We run into real problems when we *expect*, rather than *hope* to achieve ambitious goals, without stopping for a moment to contemplate the possible difficulties ahead. There is nothing wrong with having high aspirations, but we need to be realistic about how quickly they can be achieved, if at all. The Dalai Lama has said 'Holding full enlightenment as your ideal of achievement is not extreme. But expecting to achieve it here and now becomes an extreme. Using that as a standard . . . causes you to become discouraged and completely lose hope'.[7]

The effect of unrealistic goals and standards can be felt acutely if we consider a simple example. Consider two people who have to drive across London to get to work on the first day of a new job. Both live in the same area of West London, and work in the same office building in Canary Wharf. Nigel has only just moved to London, and does not know how poorly designed the city is for driving. He looks at the route planner, sees that he only has to drive about ten miles and gives himself just over half an hour. Marcus, on the other hand, has been living in London for a while, and knows that, on most occasions, it takes an hour to drive across the city. Nigel will become incredibly stressed by his lack of progress on the road while Marcus will leave himself sufficient time and will avoid stress. Now, amplify Nigel's stress a hundredfold. Imagine that Nigel makes this same mistake every day for the next 100 days. Higher aspirations could lead to this sort of chronic frustration and stress, and carry us into depression.

It may seem like common sense that expectations relate directly to stress and negative emotion, but what is not often thought about is why this should be so, from an evolutionary point of view. Negative emotions are, by definition, subjectively unpleasant. They are designed to make us invest more effort in trying to overcome the impediments to our success, so that we may switch off the negative feelings. The stress reaction brings about physical changes in our bodies which will in turn facilitate this extra effort. If a goal (like getting to a new job on time) is going to be achieved as quickly as expected (as in the case of Marcus, who has allowed an hour), there is no point in investing extra effort. This would be a waste of energy and resources. However Nigel, who has allowed only 40 minutes, will rapidly become frustrated, angry, stressed and anxious because this reaction is designed to increase his efforts. Of course his efforts cannot be increased because he is stuck behind the car in front. He cannot make any progress toward his unrealistic goal. He is in a state of goal frustration.

Now Nigel is not stupid. He learns from an experience like this. He will abandon his goal of getting to work in half an hour by car, or he will switch to a different strategy – like taking the tube – which might enable him to realise his goal. He may be less smart when it comes to bigger aspirations, however. These may be influenced by upbringing.

Some parents inculcate their children with extremely high aspirations due to their own unmet needs, and 'pushy' parents may generate unrealistic standards for achieving these goals, even in children who are exceptionally gifted. Unfortunately, there is often a mismatch between what the parent expects and the child's strengths.

The aspiration to graduate from Oxford or Cambridge may be appropriate in a child with a high IQ, and hopes for competing in the Olympic trials may be appropriate in someone who has demonstrated exceptional athletic prowess from an early age. But for many children, such high expectations of success are unrealistic. If parental love and approval is only conditional on this kind of success, this sets up a very powerful and self-defeating conflict. Children exposed to these sorts of pressures can end up believing that they must always strive to achieve perfection in order to be loved, but, unfortunately, anyone who expects perfection is setting themselves up to fail. It is an unachievable goal, and one that will lead to perpetual goal frustration.

Private boarding schools that are known for nurturing great scientists, artists and scholars can equally impress in their pupils the notion that success is everything and that failure is not acceptable. Children who are attending such schools as a result of privilege rather than talent are clearly at risk of internal conflict and frustrated aspirations. It seems logical that pupils of below-average, or merely average, ability will be at risk of depression, either because expectations are so high or because of denigration by other children.[8]

The media also affect our expectations. We are relentlessly exposed to images of body appearance and standards of attractiveness which only a rare few can achieve, and we are encouraged to look like the models in our glossy magazines despite the fact that these models have the aid of a huge makeover team. Alongside the benefits of state-of-the-art lighting, styling and make-up, the final image can still be touched up in Photoshop. Many adults diet and exercise excessively and spend large amounts of money on cosmetics or surgery in the hope that they can look like the models on the television screen, forgetting that the models may be as young as 14. The phenomenon is not confined to women – male cosmetic surgery is on the increase. There is no more tragic conflict than the one between ageing and beauty. The expectation that one cannot only achieve model looks, but *maintain* them into old age, is surely going to generate a lot of frustration.

It is not just our body image that can be distorted by the media. The media also set unrealistically high expectations of success in our work and leisure time; images of the 'perfect' family, 'perfect' relationship and 'perfectly satisfying' sex life initiate patterns of goal frustration.

Reason five: The manic defence

The experience of a cold and unloving maternal upbringing led the writer Balzac to adopt a 'manic defence' throughout his adult life.[9] He overdressed and furnished his home with a lavishness he could not afford. He had aristocratic pretensions – misappropriating a coat of arms from another family and adding the prefix '*de*' to his surname. He invented extravagant tales about how he came upon his many possessions. His literary works were very ambitious and he combined a busy life as a writer and observer with many precarious business interests. His writings were informed by a huge amount of personal research in the form of minute observations on how people lived their lives. He was not content to write on one aspect of human nature but rather chose to write on the human condition in general – his huge work *La Comédie Humaine* runs to seven volumes.[10] It consists of 95 stories, novels or analytical essays and 48 unfinished works (some of which only exist as titles). The work was the result of a slow evolution.

Commenced in 1830, by 1834 he decided to group his work together in three main sections: *Etudes de Moeurs*, 'a complete history of society', *Etudes Philisophiques*, 'the "why" of sentiments, the "what" of life', and *Etudes Analytiques*, in which all human principles are described. Not only were all his writings individually ambitious, together they represented an astonishing body of work. Yet the psychological unease that drove him to write also caused him to be plagued by depression.

People who have been victims of neglect or critical attitudes during their formative years may believe that they are inherently dull or uninteresting. They may feel unattractive inside. Fearing rejection for their inadequacies, they are often too eager either to impress people, and gain their respect, or do things to please others so that they will be liked.

It is easy to spot people with a manic type of functioning. They are 'larger than life'. Their exaggerated gestures seem hollow. Everything that manic-functioning people relate about themselves is given a heightened spin to make them seem more successful and more interesting. They claim to have skills and talents that have little basis in reality. Whatever story is being related by someone else in the social circle, it is generally the case that these people will have an even more incredible story to tell – they always seem to have done the same things, but to have done them even better. Someone with this manic defence is terrified of having his fundamental core feelings of worthlessness exposed by others.

This is an exhausting and chronically stressful way of functioning, because it is impossible to please everybody. We cannot be all things to all people. It is another expectation that can never be realised. Balzac was destined to become a famous depressive, and this destiny was fulfilled. Whether depression benefited Balzac or not is uncertain because not enough is known about his life. However, although some soul searching is nearly always beneficial, it is difficult to replace a lost childhood.

Giving up on an unrealistic dream can bring depression to an end

There is evidence to suggest that giving up on an unrealistic goal can lead to an early remission of depression. Jonathon Price and Paul

Gilbert, another key player in evolutionary psychology, have published cases supporting this prediction.[11] Here are a couple of examples:

> Betty, a 40-year-old-woman, had been told that she would be made redundant from her senior management job at a university due to a 'change of leadership', despite years of dedication to the employer. She had chosen to 'fight to the bitter end' because her moral principles prevented her from giving up her job voluntarily. She had subsequently become depressed. She was encouraged to accept that the job was lost and to focus on negotiating better severance pay. Subsequently she was able to handle the situation and solve the problem. Her mood lifted.

> Another case involved Ruth and her abusive husband. Ruth's husband had been verbally abusive toward her over a number of years. He showed neither insight into his behaviour, nor any interest in changing it. Ruth hoped, as someone with strong faith, that God would 'reach in and make things better'. Her Roman Catholic upbringing had left her with the sense that her self-sacrifice would be rewarded by some sort of divine intervention. Her therapist encouraged her to abandon this expectation and to reframe her behaviour as an understandable defeat state in the face of a stronger adversary. Such a reaction, it was explained, was instinctive and designed to avoid conflict, but her belief that she could continue to be passive in the situation for evermore was not going to resolve the conflict between her hopes and needs. She realised the futility of waiting for God to improve things and ended the relationship. Her depression subsequently lifted because she had given up on her unrealistic expectations, and no longer blamed herself for her miserable situation.

In my own practice, I treated a 48 year old man who, at the age of 45, had decided to change career direction but over the previous year had become increasingly depressed. Although originally trained as a carpenter of some repute, he had decided to give something back to the community as a social worker in the child protection department of a deprived London borough. In the very first session it became apparent that he had been putting himself under tremendous pressure to do everything perfectly. This was laudable, but, in a resource strapped environment, one had to cut a few corners and prioritise, otherwise the work would pile up. And pile up it had. He was so far behind on his note taking that he was taking files home with him and working on them in the evenings and weekends. This was having a very negative effect on his marriage and his relationship with his children. He chastised himself for his poor performance, although his colleagues always praised him. The final straw for him was a failed attempt to accommodate a child who he strongly suspected was being abused. He had exhausted himself by trying to achieve perfect outcomes in an imperfect system and an imperfect world. An outcome that was a common experience for most of the social workers caused him to slip into a deep depression. He took personal responsibility for the failure to protect the child, when events outside of his control had prevented him from doing so. As his depression deepened he became incapable of continuing his job.

Underlying his perfectionism was the unrealistic expectation that he could protect every child in the Borough, despite working in an under-resourced system. There were issues in his own upbringing – some neglect that he had experienced – that made him identify very strongly with children under threat of abuse, and this led to him working long hours, getting behind on his paperwork, and struggling to do the impossible – to ensure that every child was safe.

It was not until he realised that his past issues had made it impossible for him to slow down, that he decide to leave social work and return to carpentry. He had been trying to undo his own experience of abuse through his work in child protection, and this was never going to be achievable. Although gaining some insight into his unrealistic expectations had heralded the start of his recovery, it was not until he left his job as social worker that his depression properly resolved. This was by no means an admission of failure, as he was a respected and successful carpenter. Although he had limitations in one domain, he could achieve success in another. Not only could actualise his aspirations of having status in his work, he could also better fulfil his other archetypal needs – to enjoy fulfilling intimacy with his wife and to be a good father.

So, depression had put on the brakes and had made him abandon his unrealistic expectations – the very fact that he was becoming depressed had made him question his chosen direction. It had stopped him from continuing in this futile quest and had made him realise his shortcomings. In the end he had accepted that being a good carpenter and a good family man should be enough for him. The depressed social worker was not only happier on returning to his former job, he was arguably more useful to society, but improving his relationships with his wife and children had had the most profound effect on his happiness.

The strongest argument for depression's utility is its ability to force us to take stock of ourselves and ask: 'Why have I allowed myself to become so frustrated for so long?' If depression did not encourage us to reassess things we would merely return later to the same battle. The costs would be too high. However, if depression were to make us choose more appropriate goals, change our strategies or change our expectations, this would increase our chances of avoiding stress and unhappiness in the longer term. Depression might be forcing us to focus not on our misguided goals but on our fundamental needs, the archetypal needs that make us human. This would clearly be adaptive.

But how does depression affect a change in our outlook? Why should anyone give up on a false dream or ideal just because they get depressed? What stops them from carrying on where they left off? The answer may lie in the concept of 'depressive realism'.

Depressive realism

To quote Albert Einstein again: 'The significant problems we face cannot be solved at the same level of thinking we were at when we created them'.[6] Depressed people are relatively consumed with negative thoughts.[12] These thoughts have a common theme: depressives tend to perceive that they are in unenviable social situations and tend to focus on the desire to improve their social approval ratings and successes.[13]

Field Maloney, who is on the editorial staff of the New Yorker, quotes the scientific journalist Kyla Dunn in his article *The Depression Wars*:

> One cognitive symptom of depression might be the loss of optimistic, self-enhancing biases that normally protect healthy people against assaults to their self-esteem. In many instances, depressives may simply be judging themselves and the world much more accurately than non-depressed people, and finding it not a pretty place.[14]

Kyla Dunn was commenting on the work undertaken on 'depressive realism' – the idea that depressed people tend to make predictions about events that are more accurate than those who are not depressed. The seminal work on this was carried out by psychologists Lyn Abramson, PhD and Lauren Alloy, PhD in 1979.[15] They conducted an experiment where students who were rated as sad and a non-depressed comparison group were asked to estimate the control they had over receiving a reward after pushing a button. The reward was signalled by a light coming on, but this was not, in reality, under the control of the person pushing the button. It was the experimenters who decided how frequently the light would come on. In cases where the light came on fairly frequently, which was associated with winning money, the depressed subjects made an accurate appraisal of how much control they had had over winning, realising that, in fact, they had very little control, if any. The non-depressed group, on the other hand, overestimated their control over their winnings. They laboured under the illusion that they had more control over winning money than they actually did.

In cases where the light came on less frequently, and this involved loss of money, the non-depressed tended to *underestimate* their control. Again, the depressed students were more accurate, realising that they influenced the outcome some of the time. The researchers concluded that the depressed students were 'sadder but wiser' than the non-depressed students. This was an apparent challenge to the prevailing view, developed by the psychiatrist Aaron Beck in the 1960s, that the depressed person tends to distort reality in a negative way. He observed that the depressive minimises his past successes, magnifies his failures and is pessimistic about the future. He also generalises after one set back to conclude that he is a failure in general.[16] Dramatically, Alloy and Abramson turned this received wisdom on its head, providing evidence that it is not the depressive who distorts reality but the so-called healthy population. Here is an illustration of what Randolph Nesse, the author of Darwinian Medicine calls 'diagonal psychology' – an awareness of the positive attributes of negative mood states, and the negative aspects of positive mood.[17]

It is, however, ultimately a matter of degree of sadness and of context. Not everyone has managed to replicate the second of these findings in people with a diagnosed depressive illness, showing that, although depressed people are free of optimistic bias, they tend to be overly pessimistic about the future, as Beck's work on clinical populations suggested.[16,18] Furthermore, although not overly negative in laboratory conditions, they underestimate how well they are liked and under-recall how well they have performed in various tasks in the past.[19]

However, even if depression does distort reality in a negative way (and some would still say that pessimism about the future is realistic), the fact remains that it removes the positive self-serving biases that are seen in the non-depressed. Any unrealistic expectations of success will be challenged quite radically by depression, over some time, until a more negative view prevails. With recovery, and with the lifting of mood, a new kind of truth could emerge, which lies somewhere between the overly optimistic and the overly negative. The new truth could be devoid of blind optimism: it might consist of a more humble assessment of the sufferer's own capability, containing a more balanced picture of his or her perceived *strengths and limitations*. So, on recovery, the sufferer could realise his or her true strengths, put them in perspective, and build on them. He or she could be more realistic about the competition and the length of time it will take to reach loftier goals. As with the vision quest, there might be a renewed awareness of more fundamental needs; the need to feel a sense of social inclusion, or the need for an intimate relationship might trump the misguided higher goal – to be the best social worker, the most successful farmer, the most moral employee, the pioneering philosopher, and so on. In this way, success in terms of achieving primeval goals might become more likely in the future.

In the case of long-standing problems with insecurity and low self-esteem that pre-date depression, overwhelming negative thinking could potentially break down any defences that might prevent an exploration of these deep-seated confidence problems and their origins. For example, the gloom of depression is an antidote to the manic defence described above – one has to admit defeat. The pretence that one is much more capable, important and special than other people can not be maintained in a depressive state, and neither can the defence of denial: the hidden belief that one is fundamentally inferior to others will come to the fore. Depression exposes repressed negative beliefs in all their starkness and brutality – particularly the feeling that one does not measure up. While helping us to uncover our own emotional insecurities it could stop us from projecting them onto others. If we are busy criticising others we might need to examine our own emotional problems. It is better to be self-critical than to live a lie about oneself indefinitely. Ignorance of our deepest psychological issues will only lead to further stress and suffering in the future.

Radical versus superficial change

The main difference between depression and mere sadness is that the problem causing depression tends to be more fundamental than the problem causing sadness. Ordinary sadness is temporary, and is due to temporary goal frustration, depression is caused by chronic frustration. More fundamental errors of judgment have occurred, with far-reaching implications. Transient sadness tends to occur after a temporary setback. So, following a bout of sadness perhaps only a minor change in thought or behaviour is required to prevent the same sadness-trigger occurring again. Following depression, however, it follows logically that more *radical* and far-reaching solutions may be required to meet ones's needs in the future and stop the depression coming back. This is consistent with the 'social navigation hypothesis' of depression,[20] which is to do with discarding unhelpful old allegiances and making radically different allegiances in the future. Given that the depressed individual suffers terribly, riskier and potentially costlier options are more likely to be considered. Not only does the person who feels at rock bottom think that he has less to lose but he fears feeling the same way again.

Goal reformulations

So, to sum up, it is proposed that depression helps to remove any misguided goals, misunderstandings and false optimism that have fuelled goal frustration, and the stress that accompanies this. Low mood shifts our ways of thinking to the more systematic.[21] We stop blaming the outside world and become more introspective. The 'illness of thoughts' goes to work and later impacts on behaviour.

Option one   new goals

Sometimes it is best to give up on the goal altogether: the rejected lover gives up on being reunited; the city worker decides to buy a farm; the social worker returns to carpentry.

Option two   new strategies

Alternatively, after looking at the problem from a new perspective, the recovered depressive does not change his *goal* but rather changes his *strategy* for achieving the same goal in the future. The goal has not been compromised, but some honest self-reflection and problem solving have led to a revised plan. The aspirational architect may need to be more patient – that landmark building may be ten years away. In the meantime there will be ways to build up the studio with talent. Compromising his principles by taking on some wealthy private clients will help him to build his practice and subsidise the more poorly paid but more distinguished public projects. The actor may give up on dramatic roles, and opt instead for comic ones; the farmer may switch from arable to dairy farming; the young woman who wants to have children might look for an older man.

Option three   new standards

Another possible result of a more realistic assessment is the formulation of new standards about how well you succeed or how quickly you expect to reach a goal. This is about breaking down perfectionism and impatience. Thus, a graduate may accept that he is not going to find funding for a brilliantly original piece of research until he has established his reputation. His goal might be to win the Nobel Prize, but he may need to accept that this will take years of hard work. Perhaps publishing one good piece of research over the next year would be a positive first step. Similarly, in the realms of relationships, we cannot expect to establish a trusting, intimate relationship in just a few weeks. It is more likely to take months, and there will be challenges along the way. A writer who wants to become a famous novelist should accept that good writing comes with practice and dedication and that rejections by publishers are part of the learning process. In his book the *Art of Happiness*, the Dalai Lama stresses the importance of having realistic standards.[7] Although ultimate goals can be ambitious we need to be careful about how quickly we expect to arrive at them. The ultimate goal for him is 'full enlightenment', but he does not expect to arrive at that point straight away. The point is that you can enjoy the process, and benefit from the journey of gradual self-improvement without chastising yourself for your slow progress.

Social navigation

The psychologist Paul Watson has suggested that the sobering quality of depression makes us more aware of changes that need to occur in our social network.[20] Mild to moderate depression makes us more attentive to the quality of our social relationships, the structure of our social network, who has power, who has what opinions, how these opinions differ from our own and whether they facilitate or hinder essential change in our lives. Depression usually comes about due to some conflict – conflict between where we are and where we wish to be. 'Where we want to be' is commonly repressed, not consciously recognised. If we are rushing around in a state of stress we do not have time to think and feel. Depression forces us to slow down and think more systematically. Also, according to social navigation theory it, will eventually help us get to where we want to be.

The 'honeymoon period'

What is this life if, full of care
We have no time to stand and stare.
No time to stand beneath the boughs
And stare as long as sheep or cows.
No time to see when woods we pass,
Where squirrels hide their nuts in grass.
No time to see, in broad daylight
Streams full of stars, like skies at night.
No time to turn at Beauty's glance,
And watch her feet, how they can dance.

No time to wait till her mouth can
Enrich that smile her eyes began.
A poor life this if full of care,
We have no time to stand and stare.
William Henry Davies[22]

The following is a transcript of part of a consultation between myself and a former patient, a 26-year-old woman, a secretary from South London, who had recently recovered from a depression. She had been trapped in a destructive relationship but was now changing her life around.

[How do you think depression has helped you?] It's turned my life around, basically . . . , from being insecure, unconfident, feeling that no one else would want me out of the relationship, or whatever. I can do what I want now. Getting through that depression, and that really difficult stage in my life, has made me reflect on the important things – what I do wanna do and what I don't wanna do, where I wanna be, without anyone else making the decision for me. Now I'm making my own decisions.

Before my depression my life was crap. I just used to go to work, come home from work, make pack lunch, make James dinner, do the washing, do the ironing, have a bath, go to bed. That was my daily routine, Monday to Friday. Friday night he used to pick me up. We'd go and stay at his house for the whole weekend and sit around watching telly and doing nothing constructive with my time. And that was my life.

I couldn't talk to people. If I talked to his brother I'd be accused of sleeping with his brother, of fancying his brother. Walking to the shop –'Why have you been so long?' – when I've only been ten minutes.

Over the last month I've started going out with my friends, met a couple of blokes. One bloke, Greg, won't leave me alone. And this is the thing: I realise I'm not ugly, I'm pretty attractive really, good personality, and hopefully I'll meet someone who's compatible. But it's been great, I've been meeting people, meeting blokes, flirting a lot, dancing, drinking, just doing my own stuff basically, which has been fun.

I don't always want to be in secretarial work. I've got talent. I've got talent to do other things. My lifelong goal or, what's the word, my place in this world, wasn't to be a secretary. I've shown people my art work. I've done a picture of my Dad, and everyone's like: 'Who done that?' I say it's, like, me, and they go 'You're lying, you never drew that'. And I did. I've got an artistic talent. I'm very creative. Why waste that talent, when I could have my own art exhibition. I could probably dance in a Broadway show, go to New York. Who knows? [That's perhaps a bit ambitious isn't it? Only a very few very gifted people achieve such a thing.] My talents are art, dancing, singing, acting. Whether I make it to Broadway or Hollywood or not wouldn't bother me. Just to have my own art exhibition in the Hayward Gallery would be enough. [It's good to have aspirations but they have to be realistic.] They've got to be realistic obviously, but Pisces do have their heads a bit in the clouds. That's why they're creative. [So you think you might have your head in the clouds?] There's nothing wrong with it, just as long as you don't kid yourself that it's gonna happen. I mean I'm not sitting here thinking I'm going to go to Hollywood and be the next Julia Roberts. I mean that's just ridiculous thinking, but who knows?

I don't know if you're into Tarot card reading? A friend done my cards, and they were spot on! On my tenth card it was a change of career, and time of decision making, I'm moving out of troubled waters, more obstacles ahead but you're over the worst. These cards were done six months ago. Now I've read them recently. That tenth card, which is my final card, which is where I am now, is exactly right. It amazes me.

This particular patient took antidepressant medication to help her out of her depressed state. However, as we have learned, depression is usually corrected by the mere passage of time and during the convalescent phase of depression there can be experienced a certain relative euphoria, accompanied by more positive and constructive thinking. This can only be facilitated by avoiding any excessive demands – there needs to be a period of reflection, time to 'stand and stare'.[22] This is the penultimate episode in the story of the vision quest, the process of seeing the world through new eyes prior to the return to productive life and the sharing of that vision with others. In contrast to the darkness of depression the world seems bright, and there can be a renewed love-affair with life. Crucially, this can be accompanied by a new impetus for positive change.

Thus, with help from friends, professionals or relatives, this is a time for assessing all the possible new directions before tentatively testing. Research suggests that there is a time lag between the resolution of depressive symptoms and an improvement in functioning in the various domains of work, social relations and intimate relationships. This is not surprising given the changes that need to be made and the confidence-building that is required.

Others often know us better than we know ourselves. We may know what we *want* but others may have a better idea of what we *need*. While the jury is out on the contribution our nearest and dearest can make during a bout of depression, it is probable, though not proven, that support increases during the honeymoon period, not least because the recovering depressive is disposed to social contact. In the ancestral environment it was not only easier to take time out from normal responsibilities, but people were more inter-dependent. For this reason social support may have been given more readily. In a modern fast-paced consumerist society social support may be in shorter supply. Nevertheless, those who know us best can have the most beneficial influence on how we run our lives, and fight against self-defeating thinking. What the depressed person needs is positive encouragement and constructive criticism as he recovers.

Enemies of change

People with unhelpful personality traits or inflexible moral standards will be more resistant to change. They are probably more prone to recurrent depression, therefore. More time and effort will be required in order to avoid their returning to the same unhelpful mode of functioning that led to the depression in the first place. In these cases seeing a therapist might be helpful.

Nevertheless, there is some evidence to suggest that a close support network can bring about lasting changes in an individual's cognitive style without the need for him to attend therapy.[23] Therefore, depression may be most likely to lead to positive change if it occurs in the social conditions in which it has evolved – within a close-knit supportive network of family and friends.

In contrast, if our goals have been frustrated for more external reasons – like ignorance, misunderstanding or the interference of other people – we should be at less risk of a recurrence. Ignorance can be replaced with an improved knowledge of the relevant environment. Interference from other people can be minimised by breaking unhelpful social or work ties, or having the courage to confront others and make them more aware of our needs. We have already addressed the idea that an episode of depression will, in itself, encourage more help.

Summing up

A normal healthy adult who is not depressed tends to have an overly optimistic view of his future prospects. People in their youth often have an exaggerated sense of their own place in the world and their ability to change the world. In adulthood this rather immodest stance could, if unmodified by experience, lead to never-ending futile journeys. Although we should not dispense with all hope and aspiration, in the words of Dirty Harry, 'A man's gotta know his limitations'.[24]

We have learnt that, for millennia, people have been suffering from episodes of depression and grief, plunging into a dark tunnel before tentatively emerging from the other side. During this journey it is hoped that the majority will have gone through some sort of

One of my patients who had been suffering from a depression told me how, one day, he suddenly realised that he had started to appreciate and enjoy simple things again. This had happened when he had been driving in a particularly beautiful part of North Devon. The sun was shining, and golden strands of light were filtering through the canopy of trees above him. The sudden realisation that this beautiful scene could move him set up a chain reaction – not only did he enjoy the scene, but he was mindful of his renewed capacity to feel happy, 'stand and stare', and focus on the moment. He briefly experienced a state of natural ecstasy – a rare sense of connection with all things.

A few minutes later it was necessary to attend to a narrowing in the road. Just before the narrowing a street sign read 'Change of Priorities Ahead', which took on a special meaning for him. Any advantages that might be conferred by depression in terms of a change of direction will act over a much longer term in the lifespan of the individual than the depression itself. In other words, any improvement in self-knowledge that has the potential to improve our quality of life in the long term should compensate for the symptoms that restrict us during an episode.

reappraisal, a rite of passage, or a searching of the soul, before accepting that they need to take a new path in life. Depression may have forced our ancestors to look again at their strengths and their limitations, their coping strategies, their direction, their priorities. Most people would argue that this is always a healthy thing to do. Self-knowledge is power – if we do not know where we really need to go we will never get there, and where we need to be is not always where we want to be at the outset. Regardless of the reason for falling into depression, the journey has the potential to make us better equipped, in a general sense, for life.

If we are too busy to think and feel, to be mindful, depression might represent the first opportunity to take an honest inventory of ourselves.

What follows is a theory of how mild to moderate depression may be adaptive:

- most human behaviour is instinctively (and usually unconsciously) geared towards securing survival, maximising reproductive success, or protecting one's family members (the archetypal needs)
- even loftier ambitions, and modern career choices, are indirectly geared towards these basic goals, because achieving a higher status will often lead to improved security, respect, resources and mating opportunities
- there may be two different types of depression, with different ultimate origins: (a) depression triggered by loss, where the depressive reaction fosters an acceptance of the loss, and (b) depression triggered by goal frustration. In both cases depression leads to withdrawal from futile activity, a conservation of energy, an avoidance of harm, and a period of reassessment. Randolphe Nesse and colleagues conducted a research programme which explored the idea that loss and frustration could trigger different subtypes of depression, which present and feel slightly differently from each other.[25] Their findings suggested that social losses (death of a loved one, a romantic break-up and social isolation) were more associated with crying and arousal, whereas failure to reach a goal was more associated with fatigue and pessimism.
- however, goal frustration divides into several stages. Depression and fatigue are late-stage responses. In the initial stages any perceived obstruction to a goal activates (a) the stress response, (b) a negative emotional state and (c) a greater investment of effort

- depression is activated only when goals are persistently frustrated over a long period of time. This is like the difference between stress and strain in physics. When materials are placed under tension, they are said to be under stress. If greater loads are attached the stress increases. If the stress is too high the material goes into strain – the molecular structure changes – and eventually the material passes its elastic limit: it fails to go back to its original shape if the load is subsequently removed. Similarly, if our goals are frustrated we go into stress, and when the frustration builds up too much we go into strain. The main difference, however, is that most people with depression do eventually recover. As we have discussed, moral scruples, personality problems (like low self-esteem, or exaggerated expectations of success), ignorance of the difficulties facing us, interference from a third party (someone pushing us on when we know we should stop) or the modern societal conditions of entrapment (such as poverty or unemployment) will act to prolong the stressful situation, increase the load, and make us pass from stress to strain
- depression is needed because the factors discussed above are stopping us from giving up on the goal voluntarily. They are blinding us to the fact that the goal may never be reached, and in the meantime we are suffering a lot of stress. It is an *involuntary* break. Beyond a certain point of strain there is no choice in the matter – we *will* become depressed. The state of depression is a compulsory sentence, which works through altering reward, energy and motivational systems in the brain, and so we stop 'chasing rainbows'.[26] This means that we can conserve energy and resources and avoid any further harm
- meanwhile, our community may make sanctions that relieve us of our usual duties. This enables us to go on a journey of self-discovery. In addition, the community may become more aware of the sufferer's needs and try to adapt to them in the longer term
- depression may cause us to consider an *alternative goal*, it may cause us to consider alternative standards by which to judge our progress toward the goal (particularly relevant to the perfectionist) or it may cause us to reflect on an *alternative goal-seeking strategy* (see Appendix 1)
- depression helps us to consider these alternatives by shifting our thinking to the more realistic and more systematic. We are forced to be self-centred and introspective because social interaction no

longer holds any pleasure for us. We are not distracted by activities directed towards pleasure. Moreover, the pain of depression will make us consider more radical solutions to avoid returning to the same state of incapacity. Radical solutions may well be required: thinking along the same lines will often cause us to return to the same problems

- the advice of others is useful at this stage of reassessment. Depression would have evolved in tight-knit communities in which such advice would have been available
- the honeymoon period often experienced by people as they recover from their depression can give them the motivation to embark on radical life solutions. Things will often get worse before they get better.

References

1 *Magnolia*, film directed by Paul Thomas Anderson 1999.

2 *Jean de Florette*, film directed by Claude Berri, 1986.

3 *Manons des Sources*, film directed by Claude Berri, 1986.

4 Price J. The adaptive function of mood change. *British Journal of Medical Psychology*. 1998; **71**: 465–77.

5 Hagen EH. The bargaining model of depression. In: Hammerstein P, editor. *Genetic and cultural evolution of cooperation*. Cambridge MA: MIT Press; 2003, p. 95–123.

6 Attributed but source unknown (www.quotationspage.com/quotes/Albert Einstein).

7 Dalai Lama and Cutler HC. *The art of happiness: a handbook for living*. London: Hodder and Stoughton; 1999.

8 Rigby K. Consequences of bullying in schools. *Cananadian Journal of Psychiatry*. 2003; **48**: 583–90 .

9 Storr A. *The dynamics of creation*. London: Penguin; 1991.

10 Balzac H de. *La comédie humaine*. Paris: Seuil; 1965.

11 Sloman L, Price J, Gilbert P *et al*. Adaptive function of depression: psychotherapeutic implications. *American Journal of Psychotherapy*. 1994; **48**: 410–4.

12 Haaga DAF, Ernst D, Dyck MJ. Empirical status of cognitive theory of depression. *Psychological Bulletin*. 1991; **110**: 215–36.

13 Sheppard C, Teasdale JD. Depressive thinking: changes in schematic mental models of self and world. *Psychological Medicine.* 1996; **26**: 1043–51.

14 Maloney F. *The depression wars: would honest abe have written the Gettysburg Address on Prozac?* Posted on Thursday, 3 November 2005 at www.slate.com.

15 Alloy LB, Abramson LY. Judgment of contingency in depressed and non-depressed students: sadder but wiser? *Journal of Experimental Psychology. General.* 1979; **108**: 441–85.

16 Beck AT, Rush AJ, Shaw BF *et al. Cognitive therapy of depression.* New York: Guilford; 1979.

17 Nesse RM. Natural selection and the elusiveness of happiness. *Philosophical Transactions of the Royal Society of London. Series B, Biological Sciences.* 2004; **359**: 1333–47.

18 Strunk DR, Lopez H, De Rubeis RJ. Depressive symptoms are associated with unrealistic negative predictions of future life events. *Behaviour Research and Therapy.* 2006; **44**: 861–82.

19 Pacini R, Muir F, Epstein S. Depressive realism from the perspective of cognitive-experiential self-theory. *Journal of Personality and Social Psychology.* 1998; **74**: 1056–68.

20 Schwarz N, Clore GL. Feelings and phenomenal experiences. In: Higgins ET, Kruglanski A, editors. *Social psychology: handbook of basic principles.* New York: Guilford; 1996, p. 433–65.

21 Watson PJ, Andrews P. Toward a revised evolutionary adaptionist analysis of depression: the social navigation hypothesis. *Journal of Affective Disorders.* 2002; **72**: 1–14.

22 Davies WH. *Complete poems.* London: Jonathan Cape; 1967.

23 Johnson JG, Alloy LB, Panzarella C *et al.* Hopelessness as a mediator of the association between social support and depressive symptoms: findings of a study of men with HIV. *Journal of Consulting and Clinical Psychology.* 2001; **69**: 1056–60.

24 *Dirty Harry,* film directed by Don Siegel 1971.

25 Keller MC, Nesse RM. Is low mood an adaptation? Evidence for subtypes with symptoms that match precipitants. *Journal of Affective Disorders.* 2005; **86**: 27–35.

26 Gilbert P. *Overcoming depression.* London: Constable Robinson; 2000.

CHAPTER 8

Beneficial by-products

Leaving the evolutionary argument aside for the moment, let us consider whether there are any *incidental* benefits to be derived from an episode of depression, that are secondary to those already mentioned. If we have experienced depression in the past, are we now better placed to put life's problems in perspective, to show more compassion and empathy to others and to be more creative in our thinking?

Coping with suffering

Expecting the world to treat you fairly because you are a good person is like expecting a bull not to attack you because you are a vegetarian.
Dennis Wholey[1]

As we advance in life it becomes more and more difficult, but in fighting the difficulties the inmost strength of the heart is developed.
Vincent van Gogh[2]

In the middle of difficulty lies opportunity.
Albert Einstein[3]

It is a commonly held belief that man is on a different spiritual and moral plane from the rest of the animal kingdom. Animals are not afforded souls in many religions, but humans are. Humans are in an elevated position – at the top of the Buddhist hierarchy, for example. Many Christians continue to believe that man was created in God's image: the 'son' of God was contained within a human body. No wonder Darwin was fearful of exposing his theories of natural selection, because this put us back among the animals, with the struggle for survival being the most fundamental guiding principle above all others.[4]

Many people of faith believe that God can intervene in our lives, to cause or relieve suffering, depending on how we behave. It follows that if a man leads a good and moral life, in the face of life's challenges, this will be rewarded, if not in his lifetime, then in the afterlife. Similarly, suffering during life could be God's punishment for previous sins. The concept of Karma and the Roman Catholic confessional rituals are good examples of this thinking.

Darwin, however, has placed suffering at the heart of life. To live is to suffer, because we are all instinctively fighting against the prospect of our own demise or the extinction of our own species. Nature is characterised by competition and a struggle for survival, so to be part of nature is to be in a state of turmoil. Life is inevitably full of suffering whether or not one is moral.

Although this might seem difficult to credit, there is some solace to be obtained from accepting that one will inevitably suffer, and suffer frequently. It is better to accept suffering than to resent it. Stanley Jackson, the author of *Melancholia and Depression: from Hippocratic times to modern times* says, with regard to the suffering caused by depression, 'With such distress, we are at the very heart of being human'.[5] Furthermore, he states that it is fundamentally human to become distressed by the distressed states of others.

But can it be argued that suffering in particular is beneficial to the organism in the long term? This is a pertinent question because depression causes intense suffering. The German philosopher Friedrich Nietzsche said 'What does not destroy me, makes me stronger.'[6] Buddhism teaches us how we can learn from suffering, find meaning in it, and consequently gain strength. Thus, depression could make us better equipped to deal with troubled times ahead. The Dalai Lama states that the time and effort spent finding meaning in suffering will reap rewards when adversity strikes in the future: 'a tree with strong roots can withstand the most violent storm, but the tree can't grow roots just as the storm appears on the horizon'.[7]

If depression were to put life's hardships in perspective this could be regarded as an adaptive function. William Styron wrote on his own experience of depression:

By far the great majority of the people who go through even the severest depression survive it, and live afterward at least [my italics] as happily as their unaffected counterparts . . . acute depression inflicts few permanent wounds . . . most victims live through . . .

relapses, often coping better because they have become psychologically tuned by past experience to deal with the ogre.[8]

It is ironic to suggest that depression may provide extra resilience in the face of life's problems, when most self-help books are concerned with how to increase one's resilience toward getting depression in the first place.

A problem with this argument is that someone who has experienced one episode of depression runs a higher risk of developing depression in the future, when compared with someone who has never experienced it. There is some evidence to suggest that people exhibit a decrease in tolerance to the impact of stressful life events as the number of previous depressive episodes increases.[9] In other words depression becomes more 'endogenous' (see definitions) with increasing numbers of episodes, requiring less stress to trigger it. In severe depression the chance of a recurrence might be as high as two thirds over nine years.[10] However, the recurrence risk depends on the severity of the original depression. Most people who get depressed have mild or moderate depression, which confers a smaller risk of recurrence and most do not end up seeing a psychiatrist. The recurrence figure for depression in the general population is probably much lower.

There are some biological explanations for the tendency of depression to recur. Plastic changes may occur in the brain as a result of childhood trauma, which are then expressed in terms of psychological (cognitive) vulnerability. 'Depression pathways' in the brain may be reinforced when we experience stress. These reinforced pathways could subsequently be recalled when we are exposed to similar stresses in the future. Also, some people with very high genetic vulnerability seem to experience recurrent spontaneous depressions.

However, at the level above biology, recurrence is likely in some people because they do not gain insight into their psychological vulnerabilities, or because they have poor coping skills – they do not always learn from experience. Without adequate support and advice someone may return to the same lifestyle that made him depressed in the first place. Also, that person may fail to acquire new skills for dealing with that same situation should it recur in the future.

This does not necessarily imply that no-one with recurrent depression learns from their mistakes. Every day thousands of people are forced to return to stressful lifestyles due to events outside their control. We will consider this point in more detail in the next chapter.

Empathy and compassion

When you are aware of your pain and suffering, it helps you to develop your capacity for empathy, the capacity which allows you to relate to other people's feeling and suffering. This enhances your capacity for compassion towards others. So as an aid in helping us to connect with others, it can be seen as having value.
Dalai Lama[7]

As well as toughening our resolve and making us more resilient, the suffering endured during depression could improve our deftness in the social relationships which are so crucial to our social support and social status. William Wordsworth believed in the 'humanising' effect of distress: suffering can put us more in touch with our emotions and the emotions of others. For example, in his poem *The White Doe Of Rylstone* (the fourth canto) the heroin knows that her duty is not to interfere with events, however negative, but to '. . .abide the shock, and finally secure, o'er pain and grief a triumph pure.'[11]

Understanding the moods and emotions of others is the essence of empathy. Accurate empathy is a very useful skill for anyone to have in everyday life. It helps us to predict behaviour in others and helps us to moderate our own behaviour so as not to cause offence. Moreover, empathy makes us more *popular*. It is a feature of human nature to be flattered when someone else reflects on how we might be feeling. It reflects a generosity of spirit, a willingness to help us cope with our feelings. And it is cathartic for us to share our feelings with others, even if we regard ourselves as very private.

A person who understands the emotional lives of others is more likely to behave in compassionate and sensitive ways towards them. Even the most apparently hostile person tends to remember acts of compassion, and may, in return, offer help and assistance to the person who has shown this compassion.

Empathy is a central component of 'emotional intelligence'.[12] This attribute may be more important than general intelligence (IQ) in negotiating relationships and career progression. Due to the influence of emotional intelligence, people with high IQs can founder, while people with modest IQs can do well. Deficits in emotional intelligence can sabotage the intellect and ruin careers. They can also lead to problems in marriage and parenting. Depression may help to build emotional intelligence and in so doing facilitate more success and greater happiness in the future.

Couples can become closer after one partner has been through depression. Mutual empathy, along with mutual respect, is the basis of fulfilling intimate relationships. The lover who seeks to control the other partner through threats of sexual, psychological or emotional sanctions is too 'tied up' in his own needs to show true love. Similarly, the person who adopts a submissive role in a relationship is not always inviting a loving response. Lacking anticipation of how a partner might feel as a result of our actions will sabotage our relationships. Conversely, having the skill of accurate empathy will increase our chances of success. So depression may help our intimate relationships in the long term.

What evidence is there that depression is linked to empathy? Researchers at the University of West Florida examined 53 women with reactive depression who worked or planned to work as nurses, counsellors or social workers.[13] They used questionnaires to determine the severity of their depression and its relationship to life events. A further set of questionnaires determined how empathic they were. An association was found between the severity of their depressive symptoms and the degree of empathy that they expressed.

Buddhist philosophy attaches great importance to suffering in facilitating greater compassion towards our fellow human beings.[7] If we have not suffered in our own lives to a significant degree then Buddhist teachings suggest that we should train our minds to help us to understand and experience the suffering of others. The Buddhist practice of *Tong-Len* encourages us to take on the suffering of others actively, by visualising their agony, while at the same time imagining giving up all of our own resources, good health and good fortune. Arguably the person who has been depressed does not need to train his mind in this way. He knows what it means to suffer.

Humility

To quote the Dalai Lama again, '. . . reflecting on your suffering can reduce your arrogance and your feelings of conceit.'[7] Depression is not only humbling because it makes us suffer, but also because it makes us dependent on others to a degree; it makes us realise that we are all dependent on each other for our survival.

However, is humility a helpful virtue? The philosopher Spinoza suggested that humility was a kind of sadness, 'born of the fact that a man considers his own lack of power, or weakness.'[14] However, humility could have a positive effect on fitness by allowing us to think with reason, and avoid fighting the futile battles that we have considered in the last chapter, especially if we have exaggerated expectations for success.

Humility is different from lowliness, servility and reduced self-esteem: it is about understanding one's limitations without falling out of love with oneself. Humble people, in their appreciation of the fact that all humans are 'nearly nothing' compared with greater powers in the heavens or in the universe, feel more connected to others than do pompous people. Humility, and the self-knowledge that accompanies it, contrast with the ignorance that accompanies pride and arrogance.

Humility leads to self-knowledge by allowing us to understand our weaknesses. This may temporarily make us sad, but this same sadness, caused by acknowledging the truth about ourselves, can give us the drive to fight for self-improvement and will lead to contentment in the longer term.

Compassion presupposes an appreciation of the fact that others are just as capable of experiencing joy, pain happiness and suffering as we are – a product of empathy. It also requires us to have respect for others, a respect that can only come from humility.

Showing compassion will lead to reciprocal acts when we need the help and support of others. No-one is an island. We are all ultimately dependent on each other. The compassionate person knows this – he or she feels responsible for the wellbeing of the community because this is the same thing as being responsible about his or her own welfare.

In summary, people do not have a choice about whether to suffer or not during a depressive illness. Depression is a period of enforced suffering. The unique pain of the condition could lead to a positive transformation of character, by increasing empathy, humility and compassion.

Although this is not an argument for depression's ultimate function, there may have been incidental benefits for our ancestors. They lived in communities where their wellbeing was partly determined by social rank and the strength of their social ties. The development of these personality traits could have improved man's differential reproductive success. Furthermore, developing accurate empathy would have had a direct effect on sexual selection by improving the success of his intimate relationships.

Creative thinking

> Two roads diverged in a wood, and I –
> I took the one less travelled by,
> And that has made all the difference.
> Robert Frost (1874–1963)[15]

Bernard Berenson defined creative genius as 'the capacity for productive reasoning against one's training'.[16] Creativity finds its expression in all walks of life – from the artistic to the scientific, from the political to the entrepreneurial. It is fundamental to groundbreaking and influential forms of artistic expression. It is the 'bright idea' of successful entrepreneurs, who see a gap in the market or, by virtue of their unique vision, see opportunities being created in the future. On the grand scale of modern civilisations creativity of thought drives revolutionary scientific theories and discoveries. However, in smaller, antiquated communities a creative thinker would also have been valued. The creative thinker is often catapulted to a higher rank in society, thereby increasing his wellbeing.

In 1996 Felix Post, Emeritus physician to the The Bethlem Royal Hospital and the Maudsley Hospital in London, published a paper which suggested that depression might be linked to creative genius.[17] He examined the post-mortem biographies of 100 great American and British writers and made retrospective diagnoses of depression, using modern criteria, where this was applicable. Although he had selected the writers on the basis of acknowledged genius, rather than on any suspicion that they may have been depressed, *of the 100 writers no fewer than 50 had experienced depression according to his psychiatric assessment.* Of these, 16 were regarded as 'severely disabling depressions', while two had experienced what seemed to be psychotic depressions. If one accepts that grief may be just a briefer form of depression, then we can include a further ten writers, who fall under the category of 'brief reactions'. Fifteen were thought to have 'depressive traits' in their personality, although this concept is not rigorously defined. Great poetry has also been shown to be related to depression.[18] In a retrospective study, poets born in Britain and Ireland between 1705 and 1805 had a 30 times higher risk of a 'mood disorder' than the general population.

History is strewn with great depressive geniuses; these include the painters Michelangelo and Miro, the scientist Darwin, the philosopher Shopenhauer, the composer Schumann and the political leader Churchill.[19] So how can we explain the link between depression and creative success? Does depression cause creative thinking? Many might assume that depression would obstruct the creative process. There is a perception that depression is an entirely negative influence on success in the artistic, political and scientific arenas. However, a definite link that warrants explanation can be made between depression and creative success.

Many writers have suggested that creativity must spring from the emotional pain of depression. The eminent psychoanalyst and author Anthony Storr suggests, in his book *Churchill's Black Dog, Kafka's Mice, and Other Phenomena of the Mind*,[20] that Churchill's indomitable courage in standing up to Nazi tyranny can be attributed to his 'depressive personality'. The source of his depression is traced to his experience of parental neglect, as well as genetic factors. It is suggested that, as a strategy against this malady, Churchill developed 'extreme ambition and a pugnacious will'.

David Aubrey's book *Finding Hope in an Age of Melancholy* not only draws on history, but also expands on Aubrey's own experiences of depression, to propose that 'epidemics of melancholy' have been both a 'goad to creativity' and 'the scourge of self-delusion'.[21] In other words, the epidemic of depression that we are currently experiencing is nothing new and is not necessarily a bad thing, because it will make us face up to our cultural problems and produce creative solutions. Incidentally, Aubrey also claims that depression led him back to religious faith, and helped him to develop a greater feeling of connection with other human beings.

Aristotle distinguished between certain mental illnesses that are detrimental to artistic achievement, and those that are 'sacred' because they lead to inspiration. He suggested that melancholia could be considered a sacred type of madness because of its contribution to new ideas and philosophies: 'madness, provided it comes as the gift of heaven, is the channel by which we achieve the greatest blessings'.[22]

Anthony Storr's important book *The Dynamics of Creation*, put forward a convincing argument for the idea that creativity that can flow from the depressive personality.[23] He wrote: 'A depressive, convinced that he is unloved by those close to him, may seek to win a more general recognition of his merits by acquiring public acclaim; and producing more creative work is one way of doing this'.

However, as Storr points out, finding love in areas that are separate from family and friends is not as rewarding, in terms of repairing one's low self-esteem, as the adulation received from those close to us. Any boost that one feels to one's self-esteem, as a result of receiving a literary award, a Nobel prize or an Oscar, does not last. Feelings of emptiness and a lack of self-worth can be unlimited in depression, and they are unlikely to be alleviated by public adulation, no matter how much is received.

As Anthony Storr put it: 'However much is poured in from the outside, it is never enough to fill the aching void'.[23] This is consistent with the manic defence that causes some of us to become very successful, in terms of status, but leads to us feeling ultimately unfulfilled. We end up neglecting more important archetypal needs because of an unresolved internal conflict. Such a strategy can lead to the depressive episode per se, due to chronic goal frustration. It is well recognised that low self-esteem is a common antecedent of depression. Storr outlined three main intrapsychic processes at work in the person with the depressive personality:

- *the expression of aggressive impulses* the 'depressive' often feels hostility towards particular people in the past or present, albeit unconsciously, for the lack of love that they may have shown to him. Freud stated that the depressive person is unable to show this aggression outwardly because this may cause (in fantasy) a further withdrawal of love, and this is catastrophic to the person who feels fundamentally unloved. In the creative arena, however, there is a possibility for expressing overt aggression without a fear of direct reprisals in the form of a withdrawal of love – rather, the reverse is true. The depressive person can achieve catharsis through the expression of anger, while at the same time potentially receiving the adulation of others. Also, the aggression is not directed inwardly in the form of self-harm.
    - aggression that is particularly targeted at the past, because the past is associated with painful memories, becomes the driving force for revolutionary thinking, as described above. The rejection of much of what has gone before is, in itself, an aggressive act

– Storr reminds us that our definition of what is considered acceptable has changed due to artistic acts of aggression: the 'theatre of the absurd' aggressively attacked the narrative style.[24] Mozart strongly criticised most composers that came before him,[25] and Einstein's theory of relativity, demolished many of Newton's ideas that were previously considered to be universal Laws. The Impressionist painters, and later the modernists, surrealists, and 'conceptual' artists, aggressively attacked many of the conventions and principles of previous artistic movements.[26]

- *self-assertion* the depressive's need to ingratiate himself in everyday life, for fear of irrevocably losing love, risks a loss of individualism in his dealings with those around him, but through his artistic world he can re-assert himself, by imposing his views of himself and the world on others

- *the alleviation of guilt* depressives have a perceived need to achieve 'reparation' for past misdeeds. The depressive feels extremely guilty, feeling terrible about his behaviour, and goes to great pains to make amends, even after the supposed injured party has expressed forgiveness, right up to the point that he is absolutely certain he is still loved.

One cannot always have this absolute certainty – and this is a possible basis for the perpetual drive for creativity in the depressive – of making reparation through artistic endeavour. Poetry, for example, is often an apology for any real or imagined wrongdoings that the poet believes may have caused offence, and, at the same time, it is a catharsis. Guilt can work together with aggression. Somerset Maugham said that any novelist of merit 'offers you a criticism of life'.[27]

Some of Storr's arguments, although apparently referring to a personality type rather than a discrete depressive illness, may apply equally well to the person who finds himself in depression, since Storr himself does not appear to make a distinction. Psychodynamically they may be on the same spectrum. So, certain features of a depressive illness might heighten the sufferer's creative powers, although this could only be true of the milder types of depression. In more severe illness the lack of mental energy and drive and the lack of self-confidence are so overwhelming that any extensive creative project is impossible.

There is, however, a stronger argument to be made for the creative benefits of depression upon recovery. Someone who is emerging from the cloud of depression may feel, by contrast, a great deal of elation and joy that can kick start him or her into a creative project. Upon recovery, depressed people, who have dealt with their issues and problems, may develop a better order of priorities, a wider perspective and a more positive way of looking at the world, some vestige of which could persist beyond the 'honeymoon period' and throughout the rest of their lives. In the 1980s, researchers Ian O'Donnell, Richard Farmer and Jose Catalan interviewed people who had survived suicide attempts on the London Underground system.[28] A more positive outlook on life was often observed in these suicide survivors that could be analogous to the feelings experienced when more moderately depressed people start to feel better.

There is certainly an argument to be made that depression can lead to a greater appreciation of life, and that those who recover from depression are left with a different way of perceiving the world. I have noticed that individuals recovering from depression take more time to 'stand and stare', as Davies' poem goes, and celebrate the world around them.[29] This could certainly lead to more interesting creative work.

There is also an argument to be made along the lines of self-knowledge: depression, I have argued, leads to a better knowledge of the self and of human nature in general. This will inform any creative work.

Not all writers believe that creative thinking springs from depression, or a depressive personality. Some have argued the opposite – that creative activity leads to depression. Post describes creative labours, as 'highly intensive intellectual and emotional work', involving 'vivid mental imagery and inner struggle', and that this process , 'what shall, in short, be called "the imagination"' can 'predispose' to depression.[18] He suggests that creative endeavour results in an 'excessively high activity in neural networks', which, in turn, leads to depression. Aristotle used to warn of the dangers of developing melancholia when pursuing intellectual endeavours.[22] The humanist Marsilio Ficino regarded melancholia as a frequent affliction among people who became excessively preoccupied with intellectual topics.[18] In addition, the philosopher John Stuart Mill acknowledged that his total immersion in intellectual endeavours lead to important work, but at the expense of his emotional growth, leading to depression in early adulthood.[30]

There is a third possibility: that personality problems lead to both creativity and depression. In 1995 Arnold M. Ludwig wrote a book called *The Price of Greatness: resolving the creativity and madness contro-versy.*[31] Exploring the lives and achievements of over 1000 extraordinary men and women, this book offers answers to the age-old questions about the relationship between mental illness and greatness, and also reveals factors that predict creative achievement. It was based on over 10 years of original scientific research on major twentieth-century figures. After delving into many of humankind's greatest achievements and the special attributes and backgrounds of those who had accomplished them, he suggested that high achievers, in addition to having outstanding special abilities, also had an additional factor - a 'psychological unease', which aided the creative process. Ludwig further suggested that those high achievers without psychological problems had the natural capacity to *create* 'psychological unease' within themselves. It is not unreasonable to assume that this same psychological unease could make one more susceptible to depression than the average person.

One form of psychological unease that has been extensively studied is 'neuroticism'. Quantifiable measures of neuroticism were developed by Professor Eysenck, the man who first coined the terms 'introversion' and 'extraversion'[32] He observed that creative people tend to score highly on both measures of both neuroticism and 'ego strength'. So, if you have a neurotic type of personality, and this is combined with a conviction that you are valuable, important and deserve success, this will lead to creative works of importance. As we acknowledged in Chapter 5, neuroticism is associated with competitive spirit and success.

However, as we also acknowledged in Chapter 5, there is a link between 'neuroticism' and depression, and in the last chapter we acknowledged that high expectations for success can lead to depression via chronic frustration. Therefore, the association between depression and creativity is not necessarily causative – they could both be driven by this third common factor of neurotic personality.

The main problem with this theory, however, is the fact that not all depression sufferers, or indeed, successful people can be described as neurotic.

Conclusions on creativity

Aristotle may have been right when he proposed that high intellectual and artistic endeavour could lead to depression.[22] Alternatively, the opposite may be true – that the unease associated with mild depression may fuel creativity. Furthermore, depression may lead one to greatness through a sort of 'reawakening' upon recovery, and an inner strength, and knowledge, born from visiting the 'dark side' of existence. The very fact that someone has visited the dark side gives them an interesting perspective. However, there is a third possibility – that the neurotic personality, arising from early adverse experience, might lead to both high creative achievement and an increased risk of depressive illness.

It is difficult to prove the superiority of one theory over another. All three may be true, to varying degrees, in different people. It seems likely that some cases of depression have led their subjects to improved creative powers, and thence to a higher rank in society. However, a causal link between depression and creative thinking cannot be made in all cases of depression. It is unlikely that enhanced creativity has compensated for the costs of depression in all cases, but the propensity for increased knowledge and insight seems undeniable.

References

1 Attributed to Denis Wholley but source unknown. See www.wisdom quotes.com.

2 Attibuted but source unknown. See www.allgreatquotes.com.

3 Attibuted but source unknown. See www.thinkexist.com.

4 Phillips A. *Darwin's worms*. London: Faber & Faber; 1999.

5 Jackson S. *Melancholia and depression: from Hippocratic times to modern times*. London: Yale University Press; 1990.

6 Nietzsche F and Hollingdale RJ. *Twilight of the idols: or, how to philosophise with the hammer*. London: Penguin Classics; 1990.

7 Dalai Lama and Cutler HC. *The art of happiness: handbook for living*. London: Hodder and Stoughton; 1999.

8 Styron W. *Darkness visible*. London: Vintage Classics; 2002.

9 Kendler M, Thornton L and Gardner C. Genetic risk, number of previous depressive episodes and stressful life events in predicting onset of major depression. *American Journal of Psychiatry*. 2001; **158**: 582–6.

10 Kennedy N, Abbott R and Paykel ES. Remission and recurrence of depression in the maintenance era: long-term outcome in a Cambridge cohort. *Psychological Medicine*. 2003; **33**(5): 827–38.

11 Dugas K, editor. *The Cornell Wordsworth*. New York: Cornell University Press; 1988.

12 Goleman D. *Emotional intelligence: why it can matter more than IQ.* London: Bloomsbury; 1996.

13 Gawronski I, Privette G. Empathy and reactive depression. *Psychological Reports.* 1997; **80**: 1043–9.

14 Comte-Sponville A. *A short treatise on the great virtues: the uses of philosophy in everyday life.* London:William Heinemann; 2002.

15 Lathem E, editor. *The poetry of Robert Frost.* London: Vintage; 2001.

16 Attributed to Bernard Berenson but source unknown.

17 Post F. Verbal creativity, depression and alcoholism: an investigation of one hundred American and British writers. *British Journal of Psychiatry.* 1996; **168**: 545–55.

18 Post F. Creativity and psychopathology: study of 291 world-famous men. *British Journal of Psychiatry.* 1994; **165**: 22–34.

19 Van Lieburg MJ. *Famous depressives: ten historical sketches.* Roseland, NJ: Organon International; 1988.

20 Storr A. *Churchill's black dog, Kafka's mice, and other phenomena of the human mind.* New York: Grove Press; 1998.

21 Aubrey D. *Finding hope in the age of melancholy.* New York: Little, Brown and Co.; 1999.

22 Radden J. *The nature of melancholy: from Aristotle to Kristeva.* Oxford: Oxford University Press; 2002.

23 Storr A. *The dynamics of creation.* London: Penguin; 1991.

24 Esslin, M. *The theatre of the absurd.* Garden City, NY: Doubleday; 1961.

25 Shaffer, P *Amadeus.* Stage play, 1979.

26 Gombrich EH. *The story of art.* London: Phaidon Press Ltd.; 1995.

27 Attributed to Somerset Maugham but source unknown.

28 O'Donnell I, Farmer R and Catalan J. Explaining suicide: the views of survivors of serious suicide attempts. *British Journal of Psychiatry.* 1996; **168**: 780–6.

29 Hooper B. *Time to stand and stare: a life of WH Davies with selected poems.* London: Peter Owen; 2004.

30 Mill JS. *Autobiography.* London: Penguin; 1989.

31 Ludwig AM. *The price of greatness: resolving the creativity and madness controversy.* New York: Guilford; 1995.

32 Eysenck HJ. Allport and personality: a modern view. *British Journal of Psychiatry.*1994; **165**: 278–80.

SECTION 4

Treating depression: new perspectives

CHAPTER 9

The loss of depression's adaptive power?

The evolutionary approach to emotion has been increasingly useful in understanding the origins of mental illness, just as evolutionary biology has been useful in improving our understanding of physical disorders like appendicitis and heart disease, or physical anomalies like the 'blind spot' of the human eye. Sometimes we discover that what has previously been regarded as a disorder might actually be a defence against some other more threatening problem. For example, in the physical domain, we do not talk about 'diarrhoea disorder', 'vomit disorder' or 'cough disorder' – we have come to realise that these reactions are evolved defences. It is possible that depression may be a psychological defence against persistent stress. We have learnt that the experience of depression carries a lot of potential advantages that need to be capitalised on.

Until it was realised that the heart's evolved function was to act as a pump, treatments for heart failure or 'dropsy' were ineffective. Similarly, evolutionary psychology is helping us to determine the fundamental functions of mental systems, and whether mental disorders represent diseases or primeval defences. Sometimes mental symptoms can be either disorders or defences, depending on their context, just as vomiting can be a defence when in the context of food poisoning, and a disorder when it is secondary to a brain tumour. Over the previous pages we have seen that depression might be helpful on average. If the costs of depression outweigh the benefits in a few cases this does not mean that depression, in general, is a disease.

We need to become cleverer at explaining depression, because we are not winning the battle against human suffering at the moment: the condition is becoming more common. Although depression is not new, it is to become the scourge of the new millennium. The modern urban environment may be turning depression into something more pernicious – an illness that is more chronic, repetitive or severe due to the fact that persistent stresses are more apparent, and we have less time to think about our fundamental needs. It seems that we are not paying attention to the warning signs that herald depression, and we are suffering the consequences.

In the same way that physical pain is a warning of something amiss in the soma, mental pain is a sign that something is amiss in the psyche, which is causing a lot of conflict and frustration. If the fundamental cause of the frustration is not addressed, whether it be internal, external or both, stress will progress to depression like tooth decay progresses to an abscess. If we understand what has caused our mental pain we can then progress to address problems more enthusiastically, and focus on circumstances that we need to avoid. This means tapping into some of the darker thoughts that emerge from the journey of introspection, even if this is painful, and being able to do this with a sense of mindfulness and detachment, rather than guilty rumination. Otherwise we will become trapped.

Not only are we getting trapped in situations that cause depression, we are remaining trapped in those same situations after depression's onset. It would not be surprising therefore, if depression figures were to go up, and the condition appear more malevolent. We seem unable to take 'time out' to go on a crucial journey of self- discovery. We are not surrounded by a community that would readily understand such a course of action. Increasingly we turn to alcohol, street drugs, St John's Wort, New Age therapies or medication without getting to the crux of the matter. The modern world needs to address the circumstances which lead to entrapment – people need to be allowed to follow their instincts and find their direction. More compassion and understanding in society will facilitate this. Meanwhile the individual needs to realise that mental pain can bring about healing change, that this will lead to greater happiness in the long term.

CHAPTER 10

Should we treat depression?

The antidepressant question

The arguments I have put forward so far beg the question: 'If depression is such a useful defence why treat it with artificial drugs?' It is tempting to suggest that if we take antidepressants we might switch off a useful process.

However, we now come to another false dichotomy, similar to the nature or nurture debate that I examined at the beginning of this book; the false choice is this: 'I think I have depression so is it best to take a drug or get some psychotherapy?' From an ethical perspective, if we have developed the technology to prematurely curtail depression – a condition that causes intense suffering – it is not a trivial proposal to suggest that antidepressants be withheld, particularly as their use can significantly reduce the amount of suffering, and in some cases prevent suicide. There is little doubt that people with severe, life-threatening melancholic depression and/or psychotic depression (see definitions at the front of the book) should be prescribed antidepressants. Depression following excessive stress may leave a biological scar in the brain, which makes subsequent depressions more likely – the phenomenon known as 'kindling'.[1] It follows that antidepressants may become more necessary after a second depression. Endogenous depressions are regarded as 'pre-kindled', and more heritable – in this case a biological treatment seems necessary for a predominantly biological problem. People with frequently recurring endogenous depressions should be taking long-term preventative medication while also exploring ways of reducing stress.

However, antidepressants may be over-prescribed in the more common situation of mild to moderate depression, usually by the over-pressed family doctor. Sometimes the problems which have led to the depression are no longer present and all is needed is some time off work. When there are deeper issues at stake medication should not be used as a substitute for drastic lifestyle changes, using medicine to remove the symptoms rather than the cause. This usually brings about just a partial improvement in wellbeing, or no improvement at all, or the effects may last only for as long the treatment is taken. Any prescribing should be undertaken alongside the psychological and social changes that need to be considered. In fact, it should be seen as an aid to this process.

However, we have less support from others than we used to have. Insights that were traditionally given by the family, community, tribal healer or the local religious authority are often lacking in modern life, because of the transitory, mobile nature of community and the fall of religious faith. Therefore it may be necessary for us to seek support from a 'counsellor' or 'therapist'. There is, however, immense pressure in the modern urban environment to curtail depression prematurely and return to work. Frequently depression sufferers will not then take time to consider the psychological or social problems that led to the depression in the first place. By neglecting these issues they will be storing up more trouble for later and a condition that could have been managed by GP, spouse, family and friends ends up under the care of a psychiatrist. According to research on populations over the life span, there is a peak of depression prevalence in our thirties, but the prodrome is long.[2] In other words, there are a number of sub-threshold depressive symptoms predating the onset of the full syndrome which persist for some years. This could suggest that conflicts and issues arise long before the onset of a major depression but are left unresolved.

Addressing one's issues is not a quick or easy process and it requires 'time out'. This could be an explanation for why, if we do not address our issues voluntarily, depression will not be a brief experience. This takes us back to the issue of prescribing an antidepressant – if we are going to shut down depression early we had better be aware of the dangers of jumping straight back into the original pattern of behaviour which caused the original pain. The conclusion on treatment for depression must be that if you take a pill then you should also take some psychotherapy, even if this takes the form of a self-guided journey – a vision quest – that is geographically or mentally separate from the former life. If we abort this reappraisal process too soon it will be too easy to return to previous patterns of thinking and doing.

To sum up, the danger of only 'treating' depression chemically is that we may forget about its ultimate function. If antidepressants are to be prescribed they must be regarded as a facilitator of personal exploration, not a substitute for it. Antidepressants should always be prescribed alongside some form of therapy, even if this is self-guided, as in a vision quest, or assisted by friends, partners or relatives.

A quick word on exercise, diet and the horizon

It is interesting, from an evolutionary point of view, that mild to moderate depression, and perhaps even severe depression, may be effectively treated with exercise (aerobic, for at least 30 minutes, three times per week), given that our heritage is one of the nomadic hunter–gatherer. It is also interesting that a healthier diet, of fresh fruit and vegetables, may also contribute to the lifting of depression, given that we used to have a much closer relationship to the land. More controversial still, Darwinian aesthetics suggests that we are happier when looking at the horizon, as we would have done every day in the plains of Africa.[3] Also, people living in sunny climates all year round, like our African forefathers, do not suffer from that special type of winter depression that we call seasonal affective disorder, or SAD.

The therapist's role from an evolutionary point of view

The traditional role of the therapist has been to resolve intrapsychic conflicts arising from childhood and infancy, and this will always be important. However, the evolutionary perspective focuses, in addition, on the conflict between what the person wants, or expects, and what he fundamentally *needs*: so, the deceased will not come back to life, you will not feel more loved because you are buying a better car than your neighbour, working 14 hours per day will not bring you a sense of belonging and promiscuity will not lead to true intimacy.

If we accept the goal frustration model of depression then we should accept that part of the job of the therapist is to knock down elevated expectations, or fantasies based on neuroses and misinformation, that can never be met. The therapist needs to forcefully encourage the patient to admit defeat and give up on the unrealistic goal. The scourge of the modern age is the expectation of achieving gold when silver or bronze is good enough, and expecting to achieve it tomorrow. With such unrealistic standards, we cannot fail to become frustrated, stressed and depressed. Are we over-optimistic? Do we have what it takes? Would we be humble enough to accept defeat? Or would we go blindly on, hoping to achieve our goals 'somehow'? Case reports tell us that giving up on goals can, indeed, alleviate depression.[4]

Burton suggested, in the seventeenth century, that the key to happiness is self-knowledge, knowing our limitations as well as our strengths.[5] Self-knowledge should help us to choose the right goals, and the right standards by which to judge our progress toward achieving them. If we know ourselves – if we totally accept our strengths and our limitations – we can command more respect from others, which then feeds back into our self-confidence and self-esteem. We can plough our own furrows, without looking to others for validation.

So, the therapist should encourage us to listen to the humble assessment of depression. Upon recovery we must not be allowed to ignore the lessons that the experience has taught us. In adopting the evolutionary approach, the family doctor, partner or therapist should take on the role of 'life coach'. This does not mean telling people how to live but it does entail encouraging change and providing some objective feedback.

Above all, the life coach needs to encourage a fundamental, not superficial, change in perspective, which will ultimately come from the individual's own journey through depression – the answers are in there somewhere. The tendency to settle back into the familiar routine must be resisted. Sometimes the depressed person will be tempted to continue denying his own needs because of the pressures from those around him. He needs to break free of the shackles that tie him to the expectations of others, and cause him to satisfy other people more often than he satisfies himself. The life coach can support him in the brave quest to live his own life and not the life chosen by others. This may be risky, but the stakes are high. In the words of an anonymous poet 'Only the person who risks is truly free'.[6] The depressed individual might have found himself in an environment that is fighting against his archetypal needs – like being married to the wrong partner, or being in the wrong job – situations that threaten the unconscious drive for reproductive success.

The life coach does not focus only on internal problems – there will be external pressures to address too. A life free from depression may require putting roots down in a home, or the exact opposite. It may require moving to live in a different area, retraining, obtaining a loan for a project, paying off a loan, leaving a partner, finding a new partner, committing to a partner, giving up on a job, giving up on a compensation claim, compromising on a moral scruple, getting into new social networks relevant to a new career goal and so on. Any effective treatment package for depression should focus on defining obstacles to achievement and solving situational problems systematically.

Gaining an awareness of the hierarchy of needs determined by evolutionary pressures, as outlined by the psychologist Maslow many years ago, might help us to put our goals in the right order of priority.[7] Maslow's pyramid tells us that, for example, we should not concentrate on finding a partner until we have acquired shelter and security, and we should not focus on career fulfilment until we have integrated into a social group, or found a partner. The husband who works so hard that his wife and children leave him is denying his unconscious drive to maximise reproductive success. In antiquity these priorities were probably clearer than they are now. In the modern economy the pressure to pursue illusions of need set up by advertising and marketing eclipse our basic needs. The trend to stay single for longer, to prioritise our careers, live in cities, and live alone are mirrored by the increase in depression's prevalence. The desires to belong to a community, procreate and raise a family are shrinking in importance.

Also, to a certain extent, our goals should change with age, as we develop. The psychologist Erikson famously defined four main stages of adult development.[8] He proposed that we could not pass through the latter stages until we had passed through the former ones. So, for example, adolescence and young adulthood were important for developing a firm sense of *identity*, as opposed to role confusion. Until one had achieved a sense of identity it was impossible, Erikson proposed, to achieve the goal of the next stage – true *intimacy*. The following stage was to do with achieving generativity – a sense of being productive in terms of one's career and one's own family, and finally, when approaching death, a sense of *integrity* was the goal. The alternative was facing death with despair.

This goal-oriented approach might help to curtail a current depressive episode but, more importantly, it should help to prevent further episodes of depression. Long-term contentment will be more readily achieved if we accept our limitations, abandon our unrealistic goals or standards and consider radical life changes, where this is appropriate.

Interdependence

Hunter–gatherers pursue big game, because if they are going to expend all that energy they expect a good reward. Hunting would be very inefficient if every individual hunted down a meal-sized rodent or small fish every time he felt hungry. So we have traditionally hunted game like buffalo and elk, or caught fish in bulk. The quarry was usually too big for one family, who could not eat enough of it before most of the meat spoiled. Our ancestors had to learn how to share food, and this meant cooperation. Hunter–gatherers everywhere will act on the following logic: if you give people food when they have little and you have a surplus, they will reciprocate later, when you are the one in need. Everyone benefits in the long term, because neither party will be lucky enough to find food all the time, and food is more valuable when you are hungry than when you are full. One observer of Eskimo life once said, 'The best place for [an Eskimo] to store his surplus is in someone else's stomach'.[9] Perhaps this is the fundamental human intelligence that Lewis Henry Morgan said meets 'in the savage, in the barbarian, and in civilized man'.[10] It is at the heart of human life.

If we deny that this is our evolutionary heritage and worship individualism, we might be courting pain, stress, frustration and depression.

So, we can argue, complementing the 'life coach' approach to therapy with the 'team leader' approach will remind the depressed person to remember his interdependence. Rehabilitation should encourage involvement of those that count to the sufferer – partner, family and friends, even if they have contributed to the depression. If they are part of the cause they may also be part of the solution. Modern research has shown us that an important factor in determining whether someone functions better or worse upon recovery from depression, compared with before the depression, is the degree of social contact and support that they receive.[11] If we are depressed we need to make others aware of our needs, and in this way others may help guide us to a better life in the future. We need to explore how much our needs have been neglected by others, or how much other people have been contributing to our problems of goal frustration.

Above all, a humble assessment of how dependent we are on others is needed. We cannot live successful lives without the assistance of others. So, a balance is struck between meeting our own needs, seeking help in this crisis and, in turn, helping others. It is a truism that if we focus on satisfying our own realistic goals, and start to get results, we will be more fulfilled and will have more to give to others.

Prevention is better than cure

Although depression might be useful to those of us who are on the wrong track, it is better to avoid depression by choosing the right track in the first place. This is true at the individual level but also at the public health level.

With the exception of the invention of penicillin, history has shown us that the greatest influences on disability and death due to illness in society have been *preventative strategies*, not advances in particular *treatments*. So, the provision of closed sewers and treated water, the reduction of urban overcrowding, the first Clean Air Act of 1956, health education programmes, barrier contraception and the development of antiseptic practice, have had a much greater impact on morbidity and mortality figures over the last few centuries than the technological advances in medicine that have occurred over this time. In other words, prevention is better than cure.

The WHO tells us that depression is on the increase.[12] Such an observation does not contradict the observations that we have made so far – that depression has probably persisted in significant numbers of people around the world for hundreds of millennia – but we should address why there is an upward trend, and why depression is predicted to overtake heart disease as the main cause of disability worldwide by 2020. However, instead of trying to reduce the global burden of disability associated with depression, by just searching for ways of getting more depressed people 'treated', we should also look at the underlying cultural causes of depression in a 'sick' society, and try to put those right.

As we have learnt, depression probably came about long before we established the market economies of today. During most of our evolutionary history (99.5 per cent) we have been living in hunter–gatherer communities.[13] Only in the past 40,000 years have we been agriculturally based, and we have been industrialised for only 300 years. The slow pace of natural selection contrasts with the rapid changes in our ways of living that have occurred since the development of agriculture, animal husbandry, and civilisation. The social arrangements of our distant ancestors probably represented the best balance between the needs of the individual, the community and the environment. By the end of the Paleolithic period *Homo sapiens* was top of the carnivore food chain and was not yet suffering the arguably distasteful consequences of civilisations, including caste or class structures, power elites, armies, wars, empires, the exploitation of subject peoples and the large-scale rape of the environment. Modern civilisation may be on a 'collision course with the social needs of the Palaeolithic hunter'.[13]

Depression could be lasting for longer. This would make depression more common in the population at any point in time.

Agop Akiskal, a professor of psychiatry and an international expert on depression, observed a large group of depressed psychiatric patients over time to monitor their progress. He found that their depressions persisted for longer than 16 months in 12 per cent of cases.[14] In another study, 6 per cent of patients admitted to hospital with severe depression were still depressed four years later.[15] These patients were not representative of the general population of depressed people, most of whom never see a psychiatrist, but the high rates of persistent depression seen in a psychiatric sample may reflect a similar trend in the general population. An increase in the length of depressive episodes could be due to reduced opportunities for time out and reassessment. In other words, the economic pressures of a post-industrial world make the traditional aboriginal 'walkabout' seem like an impossible dream.

Although we like to think that we are have more freedom in the cities of modern times than when we were in smaller communities, we are perhaps less free to abdicate our work responsibilities than ever. The hunting, preparation and other duties of the depressed person in a traditional hunter–gatherer community could have been borne by others in his group until he felt better. There is not the same flexibility in the workplace today. We can argue that the freedom to withdraw from stressful situations (like an over-demanding or boring job) has become increasingly restricted in the free-market economies.

So, the main adaptive function of depression that we have examined – time out and reflection – is restricted in this environment. There are limited opportunities to disengage from goal frustration situations. Who is going to support our need to take time out for our humble reassessment? The adaptive nature of depression is presumed to be related to its propensity to make us withdraw from chronically stressful or exhausting environments. If modern society is creating novel social conditions of entrapment, it is not only creating more cases of depression, it is also preventing depression from leading to the beneficial outcome that it was supposedly designed to produce – an exit from the exhausting environment. Rates of depression will inevitably increase as a consequence. Inflexibility with regard to taking time out would cause depression to persist, and block any of the proposed benefits that might be enjoyed upon recovery from the condition.

One systematic process by which modern society might cause entrapment is through an increase in 'exclusive tendencies'.[16] An exclusive tendency refers to the unequal spread of wealth in our society; most of the wealth in many capitalist societies is held by a minority of people. A large proportion of society is at any one time in the poverty trap – where the financial benefit of working is less than the financial benefits provided for not working. Those who are living on a council estate, or 'project', have little upward mobility. A perpetuating cycle of chronic unemployment can occur in such communities. There is a lack of opportunity for quality education. The types of jobs available to someone in relative poverty are often demeaning, stressful and exploitative. Poor people are more likely to be victims of crime, harassment and overcrowding.

A major problem with the existence of relative poverty for society is the frustration, humiliation, anger and low self-esteem that can arise as a result of comparing one's own situation with the situation of others who are more affluent, especially when one feels helpless to remedy the inequity. Some societies have attempted, with a degree of success, to minimise this by physically segregating the relatively poor from the more affluent. However, apart from being morally questionable from a collectivist point of view, this is increasingly less successful as a strategy, because the modern media constantly impose images of the affluence of the majority on those who are living in relative poverty. Quite apart from leading to social unrest, this constant advertisement of inequity can predispose someone stuck in relative poverty to depression. When, despite all of one's efforts over a prolonged period, one is forced to conclude that one is not going to leave the ranks of the relatively poor, this may well lead to a depression that never resolves.

Scientific evidence demonstrates that, allowing for a drift effect (depressed people drift down the socio-economic scale), depression is most common in the poorest sectors of society.[17,18] Being trapped in poverty, with its degrading living conditions and restricted lifestyle, is a high-risk factor for depression. People in the lowest socio-economic classes are not necessarily 'poor but happy', as some people would like to suggest.

Studies that have compared unemployed with employed individuals have shown higher rates of self-reported depressive illness in the unemployed group, and the increase in unstructured time may be associated with low self-esteem, inactivity, and hopelessness.[19,20] Follow-up studies of school leavers, and large numbers of people who have been made redundant, have shown large differences in depression rates between those who found employment and those who did not.[21,22] Mass unemployment is a source of goal frustration that is highly evident across society. It is difficult to see how depression could be useful for a person who will simply never be exposed to real job opportunities.

There are many factors operating, in all socio-economic classes, that reduce flexibility in such areas as career and relationship choice. We regard ourselves as liberal and free but we must pay our mortgages and pension funds, and we have become accustomed to certain material standards of living. Bosses and partners have certain expectations of us, and our children no longer demand just attention, but also a lot of material objects that have to be paid for. Modern urban living is a barrier to the fundamental need for vision quests.

Segregating tendencies

One of the more important influences on the composition of the city population in the modern world is the need for a mobile workforce. The days are gone when people were born, raised, worked and died in their local communities. People in a modern capitalist society need to go where the work is. A job is no longer for life. Large transitory groups are created, rather than communities. The nuclear family has replaced the extended family, and social isolation is on the increase. These segregating tendencies of modern society are in conflict with one of the identified functions of depression: the extortion of a caring response from others in the community. Our nearest and dearest can help offer solutions to the frustrations that led to the depression, but not if they live 200 miles away.

The exhaustion felt by a new mother, due to the demands of labour and a dependent new-born baby, will often progress to post-natal depression if support is not provided. It could be argued that in antiquity, when there were larger family units living in close proximity, a caring response from others would have been commonplace.[23] If insufficient care had been given initially, the onset of post-natal depression would have prompted a response. Grandparents, older aunts and uncles, and others often have a wealth of parenting experience and the time available to enable them to usefully contribute some help to the mother. To a certain extent giving this help would have been instinctive – we instinctively give assistance to people who share our genes, a phenomenon called 'inclusive fitness'.[24] It is claimed that only four per cent of mothers suffer from post-natal depression in Hong Kong, compared to ten per cent in the west.[23] This is attributed to a much greater level of support, particularly in the first month after the birth, when, traditionally, all the domestic chores are carried out by friends and relatives. A high proportion of post-natal depression cases last for over a year in the west.

Depression may now be so prevalent because we are 'bereft of kin, beliefs, rituals' that routinely extricated our ancestors from futile battles for unreachable goals.[13]

However, there are also social problems of our time that help to extend depression. Professor Akiskal and his colleagues examined 137 depressed people who had not shown complete recovery from depression after two or more years.[14] These people's 'chronic depressions' tended to be 'low grade' and 'intermittent' in nature. Many cases had co-existing alcohol or drug addiction or medication-induced depression.

Of the people in whom major depression was the sole problem nearly all had complicated and unresolved social and family issues, as well as persisting intrapsychic conflicts. Examples of ongoing difficulties for this group included a succession of multiple bereavements or other losses, disability of the spouse or marital difficulties. The segregating tendencies of modern life cause and perpetuate such problems.

The media machine

The malignant force of the media machine is evident everywhere – on the train, on the bus, under the windscreen wiper, on the hoarding, on the website, covering the coffee cup and lining the walls of lifts and toilets. Its well-oiled cogs perpetually reinforce material aspirations, turning us into consumers of status symbols, making us feel lesser human beings if we cannot buy an expensive car or a wardrobe of designer clothes. The media tell us that we should all be thin and attractive, perfect lovers, perfect parents, brilliant company, immensely talented and successful money-earners. They tell us that we can all be celebrities. The language of commerce is lying to us constantly in order to 'shift units'. We need to contest the lies so that we may order our priorities properly and have more realistic expectations. This is becoming increasingly hard to do.

Hence, too many of us engage in what the influential clinical psychologist Albert Ellis called 'musterbating'.[25] People who 'musterbate' have an almost addictive attachment to the word 'must'. In their scheme of things the world *must* be a better place, people *must* do as we tell them, we *must* have what we want. Such egocentricity means that we fail to realise that our own desires often conflict with other people's needs. We cannot *demand* things from the world, because the world is an imperfect place and it does not owe us anything; it certainly does not revolve around us.

Nevertheless, we can all fall into the trap of making 'demand statements' from time to time, and we can get caught up in defending our human rights, when the truth is that one person's right is often at balance against another's. A woman might feel that she has the right to adopt a child, but if she is proven to be unable to provide adequate care for that child then adoption should be refused. The woman does not have an inalienable right to bring up a child; her right is weighed against the needs of the child.

We cannot always get a job that we have trained for if the market conditions are not right. We may have to retrain. Sometimes life is just tough. The only useful demand statement that we can make is: 'We must accept that we can not always get what we want in life'. There is a difference between what would be preferable and what we must have.

It is not in the best interests of the media to give a balanced view – between aspiration and realistic opportunity, or between rights and responsibilities. Celebrity magazines are all about the individual achieving his dreams, usually without recourse to others.

Moving forward

We can adapt our culture to minimise the risk of developing depression by respecting depression's evolutionary origins and by addressing our fundamental needs. We do not necessarily need to return to the hunter–gatherer lifestyle to reduce the prevalence of depression, but we need to understand its origins. If we know that goal frustration is key then we can keep a check on false aspirations and resist the lure of the media.

We are social animals. That is our heritage. We should reorder our priorities so that interdependent communities, including strong family ties, are valued as highly as individual freedoms. We may have too much freedom in our modern cities, at the expense of more collectivist instincts. The focus on individual freedoms is an understandable reaction to the evils of twentieth-century fascism and the restriction of liberty behind the iron curtain. However, our recent history may have caused us to swing too far away from the instinct for interdependence.

If we wish to avoid the pain of depression at the individual level, or reduce the prevalence of depression on the global level, the sooner we try to understand its ultimate function the better.

Combating stigma

In 2004 a group of researchers sought to examine public attitudes toward depression in Istanbul, where there is a high level of depression.[26] Seven hundred and seven people, who were sampled from a broad spectrum of the general population, completed the survey. The results were quite shocking. Nearly half of them perceived people with depression as dangerous. More than half stated that they would not marry a person with depression, and nearly half stated that they would not rent their house to a person with depression. These attitudes were extreme enough, but one-quarter also stated that depressive patients should not be free to roam in the community. Many of the respondents believed that depression was caused by a weakness of the personality and they expressed a willingness to isolate depressed people from the society. Needless to say, notwithstanding the high prevalence of depression in Istanbul, there is still considerable stigmatisation associated with it.

We are not free of stigmatisation and prejudice in the UK, despite laudable efforts by the Royal College of Psychiatrists to encourage more positive attitudes in their *Defeat Depression* campaign.[27,28] The campaign achieved a modest improvement in attitudes of the order of five to ten per cent. Arguably, however, the campaign medicalised the condition and further helped to marginalise depressed people. Vague euphemisms for depression are still written on 'sick notes' by family doctors in the UK; 'viral illness', 'stress' and 'exhaustion' are common ones. They are designed to protect the patient from prejudice at work, and prejudice there is, in large measure. A great number of employers continue to believe that people who have experienced depression can not meet the demands of the modern working environment.

The term 'nervous breakdown' is often used in the context of depression. The term carries with it notions of irretrievable collapse under the pressures of living. There is a sense of constitutional weakness.

Depression is, according to many, due to a flaw in the character, a self-indulgent weakness of spirit. Many people in the UK in the twenty-first century believe that depressed people need to 'pull themselves together', and stop 'wallowing in it'.

The logical arguments presented in this book reframe depression as a universal ancient and common condition. If becoming depressed demonstrates a weakness then this is a potential weakness shared by most of us – the main factor determining its manifestation within us being the chronic frustration of our fundamental human needs by our own expectations or due to influence of others. Thus depression should be regarded as a natural consequence of being a social mammal. Depressed people deserve not only our compassion but also our respect. They could be embarking on an enlightening quest, acquiring new insights, and strengths, that will be of benefit to everyone.

The evidence that has been accrued so far suggests that we need to reframe our view of depression from one of disease to one of defence. We could say that depression, in all its forms, is as much a part of human life as forming close bonds with others. A global perspective has allowed us to appreciate that this way of looking at depression is already the norm in certain cultures of the world.

If depressed people are not castigated for withdrawing from work and social engagements, but instead are allowed space and time to go on a journey of discovery, they should become stronger as a result. Nurturing someone through a depressive episode is in the best interests of society. Although the behaviour of depressed people can cause difficulty for others, the potential exists for sufferers to contribute even more effectively towards community life upon recovery than they did before the onset of the illness.

The stigma surrounding depression in many cultures is puzzling, because it is a part of life, and always has been. As we have seen, there are a great many individuals who have lived through depression to produce some of the most important contributions to politics, art, science and philosophy the world has known.

The final conclusion

While edging towards our goals, fighting long and hard against obstacles, or refusing to let loved ones go, we may become depressed. But during this journey of self-discovery we may gain important insights that will help us achieve greater success and happiness in the future. The history of humanity tells us that in depression we may find the hitherto hidden map which can help us find the ultimate treasures – happiness and self-knowledge. Depression may help us to navigate the complex world of human culture, with all its varied challenges and rewards.

References

1 Kendler M, Thornton L, Gardner C. Genetic risk, number of previous depressive episodes and stressful life events in predicting onset of major depression. *American Journal of Psychiatry.* 2001; **158**: 582–6.

2 Goodyer IM. *Unipolar depression: a lifespan perspective.* Oxford: Oxford University Press; 2003.

3 Voland E, Grammer K, editors. *Evolutionary aesthetics.* Heidelberg: Springer Verlag; 2003.

4 Sloman L, Price J, Gilbert P *et al.* Adaptive function of depression: psychotherapeutic implications. *American Journal of Psychotherapy.* 1994; **48**: 410–4.

5 Cox-Maksimov DCT. Burton's anatomy of melancholy: philosophically, medically and historically. Part 2. *History of Psychiatry.* 1996; **7**: 343–59.

6 Anonymous *Risk Taking is Free.*

7 Maslow AH. *Motivation and personality.* New York: Harper and Row; 1954.

8 Erikson EH. Identity and the life cycle. *Psychological Issues.* 1959; **1**: 1–165.

9 Wright R. *Nonzero: the logic of human destiny*. New York: Pantheon Books; 2000.

10 Morgan LH. *Ancient society*. Somerset, NJ: Transaction Publishers; 2000.

11 Buist-Bouwman MA, Ormel J, de Graaf R *et al*. Functioning after a major depressive episode: complete or incomplete recovery? *Journal of Affective Disorders*. 2004; **82**: 363–71.

12 World Health Organization. *World Health Organization: conquering suffering, enriching humanity. World Health Report 1997: Executive Summary*. Geneva: World Health Organization; 1997.

13 Fox R. *The search for society: quest for a biosocial science and morality*. London: Rutgers University Press; 1989.

14 Akiskal HS, King D, Rosenthal TL *et al*. Chronic depression, part 1: clinical and familial characteristics in 137 probands. *Journal of Affective Disorders*. 1981; **3**: 297–315.

15 Kerr TA, Roth M, Schapira K *et al*. The assessment and prediction of outcome in affective disorders. *British Journal of Psychiatry*. 1972; **121**: 167–74.

16 Clough P. Exclusive tendencies: concepts, consciousness and curriculum in the project of inclusion. *International Journal of Inclusive Education*. 1999; **3**: 63–73.

17 Ritsher JB, Warner, V, Johnson, J *et al*. Inter-generational longitudinal study of social class and depression: a test of social causation and social selection models. *British Journal of Psychiatry*. 2001; **178**: s84–s90.

18 Brown GW, Harris T. *The social origins of depression*. London: Free Press; 2005.

19 Feather NT. Unemployment and its psychological correlates: study of depressive symptoms, self esteem, Protestant work ethic values, attributional style and apathy. *Australian Journal of Psychology*. 1982; **34**: 309–23.

20 Winefield AH, Tiggemann M, Winefield HR. Spare time use and psychological well being in employed and unemployed young people. *Journal of Occupational and Organizational Psychology*. 1992; **65**: 307–13.

21 Banks MH, Jackson MR. Unemployment and risk of minor psychiatric disorder in young people: cross-sectional and longitudinal evidence. *Psychological Medicine*. 1982; **12**; 789–98.

22 Bolton W, Oatley K. A longitudinal study of social support and depression in unemployed men. *Psychological Medicine*. 1987; **17**: 453–60.

23 Hagen EH. The functions of postpartum depression. *Evolution and Human Behaviour*. 1999; **20**: 325–59.

24 Williams GC. 1966. *Adaptation and natural selection*. Princeton, NJ: Princeton University Press; 1966.

25 Ellis A. *Feeling better, getting better, staying better*. Atascadero, California: Impact Publishers; 2001.

26 Ozmen E, Ogel K, Aker T *et al*. Public attitudes to depression in urban Turkey: the influence of perceptions and causal attributions on social distance towards individuals suffering from depression. *Social Psychiatry and Psychiatric Epidemioliology*. 2004; **39**: 1010–16.

27 Priest RG, Vize C, Roberts A *et al*. Lay people's attitudes to treatment of depression: results of opinion poll for Defeat Depression campaign just before its launch. *British Medical Journal*. 1996; **313**: 858–9.

28 Paykel ES, Hart D, Priest RG. Changes in public attitudes to depression during the Defeat Depression campaign. *British Journal of Psychiatry*. 1998; **173**: 519–22.

Appendix 1

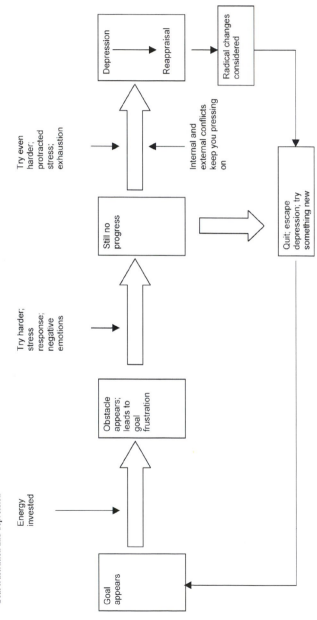

Goal frustration and depression

Index